EUROPEAN DIET
from Pre-Industrial to Modern Times

the text of this book is printed on 100% recycled paper

BASIC CONDITIONS OF LIFE

Elborg and Robert Forster, eds. — European Diet from Pre-Industrial to Modern Times

Joseph and Barrie Klaits, eds. — Animals and Man in Historical Perspective

Michael R. Marrus, ed. — The Emergence of Leisure

Orest and Patricia Ranum, eds. — Popular Attitudes toward Birth Control in Pre-Industrial France and England

Edward Shorter, ed. — Work and Community in the West

David and Eileen Spring, eds. — Ecology and Religion in History

EUROPEAN DIET
from Pre-Industrial to Modern Times

Edited by
Elborg and Robert Forster

HARPER TORCHBOOKS
Harper and Row, Publishers
New York, Evanston,
San Francisco, London

EUROPEAN DIET FROM PRE-INDUSTRIAL TO MODERN TIMES. Copyright © 1975 by Elborg and Robert Forster. All rights reserved. Printed in the United States of America. No part of this book may be used or reproduced in any manner without written permission except in the case of brief quotations embodied in critical articles and reviews. For information address Harper & Row, Publishers, Inc., 10 East 53d Street, New York, N.Y. 10022. Published simultaneously in Canada by Fitzhenry & Whiteside Limited, Toronto.

First HARPER TORCHBOOK edition published 1975

LIBRARY OF CONGRESS CATALOG CARD NUMBER: 74–18114

STANDARD BOOK NUMBER: 06-131863-9

Designed by Eve Callahan

75 76 77 78 10 9 8 7 6 5 4 3 2 1

Contents

ACKNOWLEDGMENTS	vii
INTRODUCTION	ix
The Great Hunger: Ireland, 1845–1849 by Cecil Woodham-Smith	1
Peasant Diet in Eighteenth-Century Gévaudan by R.-J. Bernard	19
Toward a Psychosociology of Contemporary Food Consumption by Roland Barthes	47
The General Relationship between Diet and Industrialization by H. J. Teuteberg	61
SELECTED BIBLIOGRAPHY	111

Acknowledgments

We wish to thank Professor Hans J. Teuteberg of the University of Münster and Vandenhoeck & Ruprecht Verlag for permission to republish chapter 3, part 1, of his book, *Der Wandel der Nahrungsgewohnheiten unter dem Einfluss der Industrialisierung* (Göttingen, 1972). We also wish to thank Hamish Hamilton Ltd. for permission to republish chapter 5 and part of chapter 9 of Cecil Woodham-Smith's *The Great Hunger: Ireland, 1845–1849* (London, 1962). Finally, we thank *Annales* for permission to republish the articles "Peasant Diet in Eighteenth-Century Gévaudan" by R.-J. Bernard and "Toward a Psychosociology of Contemporary Food Consumption" by Roland Barthes. All foreign language selections were translated by Elborg Forster.

ELBORG FORSTER
ROBERT FORSTER

Introduction

This is a collection of readings about food in history. It is not another "pleasures of the table" book suitably embroidered with French culinary poetry, nor is it another "scientific nutrition" book bearing a title such as *Animal Chemistry*, *Enzymes*, or *Metabolic Pathways*. Although social historians draw heavily on both these literatures, their task is to set the food habits of human beings in a much wider context. It is banal to say that humankind since "Dawn Man" has spent most of its time "food-getting" and "food-consuming," and for this reason alone these activities must be minutely described. More challenging, and ultimately more enlightening, is the effort of social historians to use the findings of modern nutritionists (including dietary habits as well as the actual calculation of food values) to illuminate public health and disease, demographic trends, economic and technological growth, social tensions, and even social mores, folklore, and ethnography. Thanks to modern nutritionists and to a certain imagination in the search for new historical sources, we are now learning precisely what the dietary deficiencies (in Europe, at least) were and how difficult, given the resources and know-how available, their elimination. Dietary balance, as we know, can be more important than sheer caloric intake. In any case, the problem is much more complex than either Malthus or Marx would have us believe. Nor is the knowledge gained without direct utility for those facing the horrendous hunger problem of the Third World in our time. Is industrialization an aid or hindrance? One of the selections in this book raises the issue and gives a positive answer in terms of the historical experience of nineteenth-century Germany.

Equally interesting for social historians is the relation of dietary habits to a whole pattern of folklore and culture ranging from the almost timeless rhythm of the isolated village to the rapidly changing mores and values of a whole national society in the throes of urbanization and industrial growth. In this connection, dietary history blends directly with a broader history of attitudes and values, one of the most fascinating areas of social history today. Here it joins other disciplines including human geography, economics, anthropology, and social psychology.

At their best, the historians of diet can impart an intimate dimension to historical materials in the manner of the historians of the family, the clan, the rural community, or the crowd with whom they are frequently associated. Evoking this dimension is an important part of the historian's task in any field, but it is essential (indeed it is almost inevitable) in treating an activity that is so fundamental in the life of humankind.

The four readings presented here are intended as an introduction to a larger body of literature on food in history. Although these selections by no means exhaust the many ways food can widen our understanding of the human condition, they represent four different approaches to the subject.

Closely linked with War, Pestilence, and Death, Famine has long held a privileged place among the Four Horsemen of the Apocalypse. Yet, by the end of the eighteenth century, there was reason to believe—in the West, at least—that the great famines were over. For Western Europeans, the winter of 1709 apparently marked the last great catastrophe, when entire peasant families died in their huts and whole regions were decimated by lack of food. Even the dreadful year of 1789 could not quite match the severity of 1709. It was a particular shock, therefore, for Europeans to witness another great famine in 1846 —one that attacked the whole of Ireland and has not been forgotten to this day.

Cecil Woodham-Smith's book *The Great Hunger: Ireland, 1845-1849* is a classic of its kind. It exposes the tragedy as it unfolded, a combination of dependence on a single crop, the myopia and inadaptability of the public administration, the inadequacy of the public and private response to the approaching famine, and the inhuman consequences of a philosophy of "self-help."

The first part of the selection analyzes the potato blight in "scientific language" without disguising the grim terror struck by the rapid spread of the deadly black fungus. The second part of the selection describes the futile public efforts to avert mass starvation—the soup kitchens and public works—and provides a glimpse of the human horror wrought by starvation. Were this the last of the great famines, recalling the almost forgotten plagues of the seventeenth century and the late Middle Ages, it might have passed for an aberration or biological freak. Unfortunately, it was not the last. Today (1974), from Senegal to Bangladesh, the peoples of Central Africa and South Asia stand on the brink of a new "great famine."

The second selection, "Peasant Diet in Eighteenth-Century Gévaudan" by R.-J. Bernard, is representative of a large number of studies of *l'histoire de l'alimentation* published by *Annales*.* Bernard's article has the special virtue of combining local history and folklore with nutritional analysis in order to determine what role diet played in the lives of peasants in several remote villages in eighteenth-century France. Basing his nutritional findings on food pensions stipulated in wills and marriage contracts, Bernard reconstructs an annual peasant diet. He analyzes not only its caloric, protein, fat, and sugar

---

*Cf. J. J. Hermardinquer, *Cahiers des Annales* 28 (Paris, 1970) for a complete list of articles dealing with nutrition and history.

content, but also its mineral and vitamin content, especially the ratio of calcium to phosphorus. From this, he deduces the diseases and physical defects *likely* to occur in this village population, such as poor teeth, rickets, and difficult childbirths.

Fortunately, Bernard does not limit himself to a strictly nutritional analysis. He relates his dietary findings and what he knows about the village economy to local mores, attitudes, and values. Having lived as a boy in the villages himself, Bernard brings an intimate reality to his analysis and suggests plausible, if not incontestable, links between chronic undernourishment and folklore. He evokes the ceremonial slaughter of the pig, the meticulous conservation of every edible part, from the brains to the intestines, the flow of wine at the village fête, the conceptions at Christmas, the deaths of late winter and the births of full summer—in short, the timeless rhythm of rural life. Not all practitioners of dietary history are so successful at blending caloric calculations with the "groaning beams of the peasant cottage in a winter storm." This is *Annaliste* history at its best.

Food, writes Roland Barthes, "is not only a collection of products that can be used for statistical or nutritional studies. It is also . . . a system of communication, a body of images, a protocol of usages, situations, and behavior." In this third selection, "Toward a Psychosociology of Contemporary Food Consumption," Barthes suggests that food, especially for those happy few who have enough of it, is "highly structured." The labels given to each food and the use of the terms in a social context is a "sign" beckoning like a newly unlocked door toward unexpected relationships. From fairly simple correspondences such as the apparent preference of lower-income groups for sweet foods and upper-income groups for bitter foods, Barthes proceeds to much more subtle relationships by a semantic, rather than a strictly empirical, procedure. Relying heavily on modern advertising techniques, he uncovers a whole spectrum of areas where the nomenclature of foods serves as an indicator of the entire culture. Much more than simply a means of bodily

INTRODUCTION   xiii

subsistence, food becomes an intimate part of the protocol of modern social life. "Food is an organic system, organically integrated into a specific type of civilization." Perhaps only a French linguistic scholar would have put it precisely this way.

The last selection is a substantial part of the recent book by H. J. Teuteberg and G. Wiegelman on the dietary revolution brought on by industrialization in nineteenth-century Germany. In this chapter ("The General Relationship between Diet and Industrialization"), Teuteberg, writing alone, probes the complex effects of urbanization and commercialized agriculture, especially on the new factory worker. He shows that the loss of the family garden plot did not necessarily mean a less varied diet; on the contrary, factory workers usually had a wider choice of foods in the new city market. Unfortunately, throughout most of the nineteenth century, their wages were not high enough to permit them a sufficient quantity of the new "luxury foods" (meat, milk, eggs, coffee, fresh fruits and vegetables) to replace the monotonous old staples (cereals and potatoes). Moreover, the new factory hours forced the female factory workers to rush home and hastily prepare the midday meal for the entire working family, resulting in further deterioration of the quality of food consumed. No *simple* Marxist theory of the exploitation of labor explains the deterioration of working-class living standards in the early nineteenth century.

However, in the last third of the century, the agricultural and transportation revolutions, together with decisive mass innovations in food processing and preservation—especially in canning—reversed the downward trend, and working-class diets began to improve dramatically. The technological breakthrough was accompanied by a waning of older habits and traditions of eating—familial and religious—in the generation before 1914. In the long run, according to Teuteberg, industrialization disproved both Malthus and Marx and furnished German workers in 1914 with a varied diet richer in proteins, minerals, and vitamins than ever before. In retrospect, the rural diet (dark bread and potatoes) should no more be idealized than other aspects of the life of the village laborer. By the first half of the twentieth century, the urban worker, whatever his other problems, was approaching the "freely chosen diet of the upper classes." Contrasted with the Great Famine of Ireland and the chronic malnutrition of Bernard's French villages, Teuteberg's history of nutrition in nineteenth-century Germany gives a breath of hope to the undernourished majority of mankind in our own time.

The Great Hunger: Ireland, 1845–1849

CECIL WOODHAM-SMITH

[The Potato Blight]

It is now known that blight is caused by a fungus named *Phytophthora infestans*.* It was not a sickness of the plants themselves which turned the potato fields of Ireland black almost overnight. Invasion by a microscopic living organism took place, an organism able to reproduce itself with lightning speed and "an addition to the known flora of Europe and a part of the creation which had never been catalogued before."

Blight is with us still. Every year since 1845, in potato fields throughout the northern hemisphere, the blight fungus has been present, waiting only for the right weather conditions to multiply with fearful rapidity, as again happened, with exceptional severity, in 1958.

Up to 1939 blight is estimated to have cost the United Kingdom an average of five million pounds a year. In a bad year—

SOURCE: Chapter 5 and pp. 177–183 of chapter 9 of *The Great Hunger* by Cecil Woodham-Smith. Copyright © 1962 by Cecil Woodham-Smith. Reprinted by permission of Harper & Row, Publishers, Inc., New York, and Hamish Hamilton, Ltd., London.

*For the material in this chapter I am indebted to the kindness and patience of Mr. Geoffrey Samuel, late of the Agricultural Research Council, and for the historical aspects to Mr. E. C. Large of the Plant Pathology Laboratory, who has generously allowed me to make a free use of the facts in his remarkable book *The Advance of the Fungi*. I should also like to thank Dr. N. Robertson of the University of Hull for his valuable suggestions.

1879 for instance—potatoes worth six million pounds were destroyed in Ireland alone. In the United States during the severe attack of 1928 a single state, the state of New York, lost thirteen million bushels.

Where the potato blight originated and how it came to Europe is a mystery. Early botanists and natural historians do not mention any disease resembling blight, and potatoes had been grown in most European countries for nearly two hundred years before blight appeared. A potato disease identical with blight was found in North Germany near Hanover about 1830, but the first fully recorded outbreak took place in the New World in 1842, when potatoes along the Atlantic coast of North America, from Nova Scotia to Boston, were destroyed. This attack was followed, in Europe, by the serious outbreak of 1845 and the total loss of 1846.

It has been proved that the organism of the blight fungus is so sensitive to heat and drought that its spread, for any considerable distance, by air currents is impossible, and the blight fungus almost certainly reached Europe in a diseased tuber, carried in a ship from North America. When this took place is not known, but the description of blight in Germany about 1830 disposes of a pleasing theory, that blight had to wait for the coming of steam to cross the Atlantic. It had been argued that potatoes stored in the hold of a sailing-ship became so warm during the slow passage through the Doldrums that the fungus was killed, whereas the shorter passage, by steam, allowed it to survive. But the first crossing of the Atlantic by a steamship was not accomplished until 1838, eight years after blight was observed in Germany; and early steamships, owing to their extravagant consumption of fuel, were not used to any extent as cargo vessels for more than fifteen years after the initial crossing.

Blight is now treated by spraying with copper compounds, such as Bordeaux mixture, the compound of copper sulphate and quicklime first used in the vineyards of France against *Peronospora*, the deadly fungus of the vines. Potato crops attacked or threatened by blight are nowadays sprayed on a large scale, frequently from aeroplanes and helicopters, and though blight remains the most serious plant pestilence in the northern hemisphere complete destruction of a crop no longer takes place.

In 1846, however, there was no notion of treating or protecting potato plants, nor any comprehension of the nature of blight. More than fifteen years were to pass before blight was acknowledged to be the work of a fungus and nearly forty before, in 1885, Bordeaux mixture was first used.

Yet almost as soon as blight appeared the truth was discerned; what was lacking was proof.

In the summer of 1845 the Reverend M. J. Berkeley, a country clergyman, perpetual curate of the parishes of Wood Newton and Apethorpe, in Northamptonshire, observed that whenever the mysterious new disease attacked the potato plants in his parish a tiny growth, a minute fungus, was invariably to be found on the blighted parts of leaves and tubers. Mr. Berkeley was no ordinary country parson. A gentleman "eminent in his knowledge of the habits of fungi," he had done valuable work on molluscs, seaweeds and algae when a curate at Margate, and been responsible for the volume on fungi in Smith's famous *English Flora*, published in 1836.

Mr. Berkeley was in the habit of corresponding with a French botanist of eminence, Dr. Montagne, originally a surgeon in the Napoleonic army who had become an authority on mosses and lichens. When blight appeared in France, Dr. Montagne also observed the tiny growth, and communicated with Mr. Berkeley; drawings and descriptions were exchanged, and the growth in England and the growth in France proved identical. On August 30, 1845, at a meeting of the Société Philomatique, in Paris, Dr. Montagne described the growth and claimed the discovery of a new species of fungus. The claim was recognized and accepted.

Mr. Berkeley now went further. In January, 1846, after the first failure, he published an article in the *Journal of the Horticultural Society* of London, entitled "Observations, Botanical and Physiological, on the Potato Murrain," in which, after describing the new fungus, he asserted that it, and it alone, was the cause of the recent potato pestilence. The disease known as blight, he declared, was caused by the growth of the fungus, as a parasite, on the potato plant, and by nothing else.

Vehement controversy followed. Mr. Berkeley's theory, the "fungal theory," as it was called, contradicted the doctrines generally held at that time, and many scientists, including Dr. Lindley, the well-known editor of the *Gardeners' Chronicle*, disagreed. A prolonged altercation followed, and Dr. Lindley and Mr. Berkeley argued hotly, week after week, in the columns of the *Horticultural Journal* and the *Gardener's Chronicle*.

It was generally believed then that fungi were the consequence, not the cause, of decay. Because they were usually to be found on rotting matter it was argued that fungi appeared as a result of the heat and fermentation which accompany the process of decomposition; and there was also a lingering belief that the fermentation and heat of decomposition could somehow generate life, that overripe cheese could generate mites and bad meat blowflies. An earlier generation had believed that old rags and stale cheese, shut up together in a box, could produce mice, and though scientists had discarded these fables more than a century ago, they still believed that such rudimentary forms of life as fungi could be produced by the process of decomposition.

Therefore, though Dr. Lindley, too, had observed the invariable presence of the tiny fungus on blighted plants, he had passed it over as being a normal consequence of decay, or of the "wet putrefaction" and "dropsy" which, in his opinion, were the cause of blight.

Moreover, Mr. Berkeley was now asked some very awkward questions. Mr. Berkeley's theory, the "fungal theory," must depend on the order in which the fungus and the blight appeared, and if the fungus caused blight, it must come first; could Mr. Berkeley prove this? Could he demonstrate that healthy plants were attacked by the fungus and then developed blight? It was admitted that the fungus was invariably to be found on the blighted parts of leaves and tubers, but that fact proved nothing, except its close association with decay, which was already known.

There was another important question. If a fungus was responsible, how was it that potatoes not yet dug and still in the ground were found to be blighted? True, certain species of fungi had airborne spores, and might spread from leaf to leaf of the potato plants, but how could tubers, which were underground, be affected?

To these and other questions Mr. Berkeley could give no satisfactory answer; though with a flash of genius he had divined the truth, he had little evidence to support his theory, and the "Observations," now regarded as a landmark in botanical history, which he published in the *Journal of the Horticultural Society* were almost universally rejected.

Unfortunately Mr. Berkeley never did produce proof, and the truth of the fungal theory was established very slowly, over more than three-quarters of a century. While mycology, the science of the fungi, made notable advances in the fifty years following 1845, and the life cycles of *Rust*, the fungus of wheat, and *Oidum*, the fungus of vines, were traced and a remedy brought within sight; the life cycle of the potato fungus remained a mystery. It was not until well into the twentieth century that after "one of the longest games of hide-and-seek in natural history," the enigma was solved and the habits, the method of functioning and the manner in which *Phytophthora infestans* survives and propagates itself became known.

By a stroke of poetic justice it was in Ireland that much of the final research was carried out, by Professor Paul Murphy, a Kilkenny man, at the Albert Agricultural College, Glasnevin, Dublin.

Phytophthora infestans first makes its appearance as a minute, whitish growth, resembling a fringe, just visible to the naked eye, surrounding the blighted and decaying parts on the leaves of infested potato plants. Under the microscope, this "down" is seen to be made up of countless long, slender, branching filaments, each carrying at its tip a minute pear-shaped swelling. The filaments are, in fact, fungus-tubes, and the pear-shaped swelling each carries is a container, like a capsule, which contains the spore of the fungus. The blight fungus consists of these fungus-tubes; they form a vegetable organism of great destructive power, without roots, without flowers, without any differentiation between stem and leaves, which grows and develops within the plant, and, by means of the spore container, is able to propagate itself with frightening rapidity. The spores formed on a single potato plant which has been invaded by the blight fungus can, if weather conditions are favourable, infect many thousands of other plants in a few days.

The spore containers grow at the ends of the fungus-tubes, like fruits on a branch, until they are mature, when they become separated. The lightest breeze detaches them; the gentlest rain or dew washes them off. Countless thousands then fall to the ground; other myriads become airborne, and drift.

When an airborne spore container drifts on to the leaf of a potato plant it settles and, given one necessary condition, germinates at once. The necessary condition is moisture. The spore of the blight fungus is water-borne; when it moves it swims and, therefore, to germinate effectively it needs a drop of moisture. The scientists of 1846 who attributed blight to the wetness of the summer were very nearly right. Though rain and damp are not the cause of blight, without them the fungus does not multiply rapidly. Consequently, in a dry summer there is little blight, and the fungus, though present, is more or less dormant; while during a damp season blight is at its most vigorous. Violent driving rain does not provide the conditions most favourable to the spread of blight; in gales of rain the down-like fringe, consisting of thousands upon thousands of fungus-tubes, is washed off. It is when the atmosphere is moist and muggy that spore production reaches its height, and the blight fungus spreads with such rapidity that potato fields seem to be ruined overnight. The soft, warm climate of Ireland, particularly in the west, with its perpetual light rains and mild breezes, provides ideal conditions for the spread of the fungus, and has been truly described as a forcing-house for blight.

Given adequate moisture, the container proceeds surprisingly to germinate in two different ways. Sometimes it germinates as one unit, sending a single germ-tube instantly into the potato leaf, sometimes its contents split up within the container and become from six to sixteen smaller spores, which are then released in a swarm. Under the microscope these spores can be seen, at the moment of release, jostling each other, "much more like little uni-cellular animals let out of a bag than anything one might expect to find in the vegetable kingdom." The tiny spores are called zoospores, meaning that they are able to move; after liberation they swim away and, settling on a fresh part of the leaf, each sends out a minute germ-tube to invade the leaf, but at six to sixteen points instead of one.

In a short time the leaf is overrun by a system of radiating fungus-tubes, pushing their way through, to emerge in due course, each bearing at its tip the pear-shaped containers which, in a very few hours, will release fresh hordes of spores. In this process the potato plant is destroyed. As the fungus-tubes, whether originating from large or small spores, work their way through the leaf, lengthening and branching, they leave ruin behind, the juices of the leaf are drained and the tissues exhausted; a change takes place in the matter of which the leaf is composed, fermentations appear, followed by discoloration and mortification; finally, the entire foliage of the potato plant turns black, withers, and dies. Yet this process is not purely destructive; it is from the fermentation and decay of the leaf that the fungus extracts its nourishment, the "protoplasm," or vital substance, which enables the fungus-tubes to live.

The unfortunate potato plant is now not only being devoured but choked as well. "If a man," writes Mr. E. C. Large, "could imagine his own plight, with growths of some weird and colourless seaweed issuing from his mouth and nostrils, from roots which were destroying and choking both his digestive system and his lungs, he would then have a very crude and fabulous, but perhaps an instructive, idea of the condition of the potato plant. . . ."

Meanwhile, beneath the ground, the blight fungus is attacking the potatoes themselves. How this happens was for many years one of the major mysteries of blight. It used to be thought that the disease travelled down the stem of the plant to the tubers, and one of the earliest treatments for blight, still occasionally practised today, was to cut off the stems and foliage of infected plants, close to the ground. But this operation by no means invariably prevents infection, and if done too early it may prove as ruinous as blight itself. Once stems and foliage are amputated, none of the food material which the plant derives from the green chlorophyll in the leaves can pass down to the tubers, growth stops, and the result is a useless crop of wizened, dwarfed potatoes the size of walnuts.

It has now been established that blight penetrates the soil to the tubers. Moisture is, once more, the deciding factor; if rain is sufficiently heavy and continuous, some of the myriads of spore containers which fall to the ground are washed down, through the soil, on to the potatoes. The process of destruction which took place on the leaf is now repeated: the spore container germinates, each spore, whether entire or the result of splitting up, sends a germ-tube into the tuber and the fungus then works its way from cell to cell. Blackened and decomposing patches appear on the skin of the potato and in its flesh, and eventually the exhausted tissues collapse into pulp.

As a rule, however, blight fungus remains inactive for a considerable period when it has entered the potato; only a discoloration of the skin betrays the presence of the fungus within, and such infected tubers are the means by which blight is most commonly spread. If tubers containing the dormant blight fungus are planted either accidentally or because the importance of the partial infection is not realized, as happened in Ireland in 1845-46, a small number will throw up shoots early in the season; these are infected with blight when they appear. A fungus-tube from within the potato has grown up inside the stem of the shoot, and thus, at the beginning of the season, a nucleus of infection is established, ready to develop with lightning rapidity when the weather becomes warm and moist in July, August, or September.

The Ministry of Agriculture in London forecasts the onset of blight each year from a study of the weather records. As soon as conditions favouring blight occur, warnings are issued recommending potato growers to spray their crops.

The blight fungus also infects potatoes after digging, a source of despair and bewilderment in 1845. The top and foliage of a plant can be destroyed by blight while the potatoes in the ground beneath may be sound: either the potatoes were too well-covered with earth for the blight spore to reach them or, as was frequently the case in Ireland, rain was light and did not wash the spore containers down through the soil. But, even so, danger of infection is not over; countless thousands of live spore containers are on the leaves of surrounding plants, and as the potatoes are dug they are showered with spores. If the weather is dry no harm is done, but if it is moist the spore containers find the drop of water they must have to germinate, and within a few hours the fungus is active, growing rapidly through the tubers. In a few weeks the potatoes which were sound when dug are a mass of rottenness.

In 1845 much of the infection occurred after the potatoes were dug. In 1846 rain was exceptionally heavy, the spore containers were washed down on to the tubers, which were then devoured by the fungus and became rotten in the ground.

The life of the blight fungus is short. If the air is dry the spore containers carried at the end of each fungus-tube live for only a few hours; if the weather is damp, and the spore germinates, the new germ-tube must penetrate a leaf quickly, or it dies. When cold weather comes, the work of destruction being completed, the fungus dies.

For long it remained a mystery how the fungus survives the winter and starts its work of destruction again the following year. It has never been proved that the spore of the blight fungus can survive the winter in European soil, but it appears that the fungus survives from season to season, lying dormant in the slightly diseased potatoes which are occasionally planted, through ignorance or accident, with healthy tubers. The fungus grows up within the stem, diseased shoots develop, and as soon as conditions of weather and temperature are favourable the fungus begins to form its spores again. Once spore production has started the blight fungus can spread with astonishing rapidity. In moist, warm conditions one diseased plant within a day or two releases several million spores, each one of which is capable of dividing within itself and producing a swarm of smaller spores. If a number of slightly diseased seed potatoes have been planted in different places, and diseased shoots appear in any quantity, blight can become general in a few weeks. Countless millions of spore containers germinate hourly; germ-tubes work their way into leaf and tuber, reducing green and healthy plants to decay; fields are seen to turn black, tubers, hastily dug, collapse into stinking masses, and the fearful stench of decomposition hangs over the land.

In Ireland in 1846 conditions favoured the spread of the blight fungus to an extent which has not been recorded before or since. There had been an outbreak of blight the previous year, and very many slightly diseased potatoes had been planted in the fields, sending up diseased shoots. The weather of 1846 was wet—"continual rain" yet warm; on June 6 *The Times* recorded a heat wave. Ignorance was complete; blight was not known to be a fungus; treatment with Bordeaux mixture was not attempted for nearly forty years.

The great Irish failure of 1846 is the classic example of an outbreak of blight, and the people of Ireland, gazing over their blackened fields, despaired. They were already exhausted. What resources they possessed had been used up, and death from starvation was not a possible but an immediate fate.

Once more, the question so frequently asked in the past was on every lip—what would the British Government do to save Ireland?

[Relief Measures]

The introduction of soup was greeted at first with enthusiasm. "Of all the remedies to avert the horrors of starvation, none has equalled the establishment of soup kitchens," wrote a Commissariat officer at the end of January; and Colonel Jones told Lord John Russell that "the small amount of nourishment has a very great effect on the famished individuals whose stamina are thus partially revived," adding that soup kitchens "have the advantage of bringing to our aid the active assistance and benevolence of the other sex."

Good soup, if accompanied by a piece of bread or a meal-cake, was of value, and private persons, often of moderate means, kept hundreds of people alive by distributing it.

Much of the soup, however, was not so much soup for the poor as poor soup. At Vicarstown, Queen's County, the estate of the Right Hon. James Grattan, son of the great Henry Grattan, 30 gallons, or 120 quarts, of soup were made fcr well under 1d. a quart on January 18. The ingredients were one oxhead, without the tongue, 28 lb. turnips, 3½ lb. onion, 7 lb. carrots, 21 lb. pea-meal, 14 lb. Indian corn-meal, and the rest water. The local schoolmaster described the mixture as a "vile compound," and the people, after one trial, refused to accept it, declaring it gave them "bowel complaints."

Equally economical was the soup made by Mrs. Neale, wife of Sir Richard Bourke's bailiff, at Castleconnel, County Limerick. On January 23 she used 30 lb. beef, 8 lb. barley, 8 lb. steeped peas, 2 stone turnips, 5d. worth of "leeks and other vegetables," and 190 quarts of water.[1]

Alexis Soyer, the famous French chef of the Reform Club, had created a sensation in London by composing recipes for soup costing three farthings a quart, and distributing it, daily, to two or three hundred of the London poor. His recipes were alarmingly economical. Recipe No. 1, which, Soyer asserted, "has been tasted by numerous noblemen, members of Parliament and several ladies . . . who have considered it very good and nourishing," used ¼ lb. of leg of beef, costing 1d., to 2 gallons of water, the other ingredients being 2 oz. of dripping: ½d.; 2 onions and other vegetables: 2d.; ½ lb. of flour, seconds: ¼d.; ½ lb. pearl barley: 1½d.; 3 oz. salt and ½ oz. brown sugar; total

---

1. Capt. Haymes to Routh, January 27, 1847, Comm. Corr. II, p. 27. Lord John Russell, H of C, January 25, 1847, Hansard, Vol. 89, p. 435. Grattan Bellew Papers, N.L.I. MSS. Correspondence of Sir Richard Bourke Thornfield, Castleconnel, N.L.I. MSS.

cost: 1s. 4d. Recipe No. 2 was even cheaper—100 gallons could be made for under £1, including an allowance for fuel.

"Medico," however, writing to the Press from the Athenaeum, described Soyer's recipes as "preposterous." "The debilitating effects of a liquid diet are so well known to the medical officers of our hospitals, prisons and other public establishments that it is unnecessary to dwell on the subject." Any person "in the slightest degree acquainted with the elements of organic chymistry" could see, at a glance, that the soup was "utterly deficient in the due supply of those materials from which the human frame can elaborate bones, tendon, blood, muscle, nervous substance, etc."[2]

This was confirmed in Ireland; Mr. Bishop, Commissariat officer in west Cork, complained in a letter that soup "runs through them without affording any nourishment," while a doctor in the starving town of Skibbereen had told him it was "actually injurious" to the very large number of people who were suffering from dysentery.

Soup, wrote Mr. Dobree, from Sligo was "no working food for people accustomed to 14 lb. of potatoes daily"; and the appearance of the people soon betrayed the disastrous effects of a soup diet.[3] Nevertheless, Soyer's claim that a meal of his soup once a day, together with a biscuit, was sufficient to sustain the strength of a strong and healthy man, was too tempting for the British Government to ignore. After all, Soyer enjoyed immense prestige; he was perhaps the most famous chef in Europe, and at the request of the Lord-Lieutenant he was invited to come to Dublin, install boilers, and superintend his scheme for the mass distribution of soup. "Soyer is on his way," wrote Routh to Trevelyan on February 22.

Soyer's new model soup kitchen was constructed in front of the Royal Barracks in Dublin and opened on April 5. It was a wooden building, about 40 feet long and 30 feet wide, with a door at each end; in the centre was a 300-gallon soup boiler, and

2. *The Times*, February 18, 24, and 25, 1847.
3. A. C. G. Bishop to Routh, February 7, 1847, T 64/362 A. Dobree to Trevelyan, March 1, 1847, Comm. Corr. II, p. 195.

a hundred bowls, to which spoons were attached by chains, were let into long tables. The people assembled outside the building, and were first admitted to a narrow passage, a hundred at a time; a bell rang, they were let in, drank their soup, received a portion of bread, and left by the other door. The bowls were rinsed, the bell rang again, and another hundred were admitted. Sir John Burgoyne disapproved—it was a mistake, he wrote, to feed the destitute like wild animals.

But the people of Dublin were starving, and they crowded to the kitchen; 5,000 rations had been considered the probable maximum, but 8,750 were supplied daily. Soyer's model kitchen was finally bought by Government and handed over to the Relief Committee of the South Dublin Union.[4]

Food had now risen so high in price that reports from Commissariat officers in February described "women and children returning home sobbing with grief at the insufficient food they have been able to procure with the wages of their husband and father"; the officers, wrote Trevelyan, told him they could "bear anything but the ceaseless misery of the children."[5]

The demand for soup became impossible to satisfy. In west Cork, for instance, towards the end of January, 17,000 pints of soup were being distributed daily under the Soup Kitchen Act, and about 14,000 daily by the Cork Auxiliary Committee of the Society of Friends. But, wrote Mr. Bishop, of the Commissariat, not a tenth of the destitute population could be supplied—it was "a mere drop in the ocean." Crowds waited, hour after hour, at the distributing centres, sometimes all night, and savage struggles took place when distribution began. Colonel Douglas, the Relief Inspector, reporting on the Clonmel soup kitchen, broke off to write *"I have witnessed such scenes. . . ."*[6]

February was the worst month of the terrible winter. Board of

---

4. Routh to Trevelyan, February 22, 1847, T 64/362 A. *The Times,* April 7, 1847. Sir John Burgoyne to Trevelyan, April 21, 1847, T 64/363 B. Helen Morris, *Portrait of a Chef. The Life of Alexis Soyer* (1938), pp. 78 and 79.

5. Trevelyan to Mr. Jones Loyd, February 1, 1847, Comm. Corr. II, p. 49.

6. A. C. G. Bishop to Trevelyan, January 29, 1847, Comm. Corr. II, p. 30. *Transactions,* Appendix III, p. 181. Col. Douglas to Trevelyan, January 27, 1847, T 64/362 A.

Works' inspectors reported heavier falls of snow and fiercer gales; roads became impassable, carts could not travel, horses sank in drifts and had to be dug out, the streets of towns and villages became "full of starving paupers." Not only in Connaught and Munster but in Ulster destitution increased daily. "Mobs of men and women imploring employment assail you on the road," wrote Captain Glascock, an inspector from Armagh. Families without food or fuel took to their beds, and "very many perished unknown." "People sink," wrote Mr. Bishop; "they have no stamina left, they say 'It is the will of God' and die."[7]

The period during which the public works were to begin closing down started in February, but the severity of the weather sent fresh masses of destitute surging on the works, and applications for employment rapidly increased. In Galway, on February 6, applications "exceeded by many hundreds any previous demand." In Meath, one of the more prosperous midland counties, lists were increasing "by 100 names a day." In Leitrim, 600 new names were brought forward in 24 hours.[8]

On February 4, in the House of Commons, Lord George Bentinck, an extreme Tory, proposed a Bill to spend sixteen million pounds on building railways in Ireland. There were at the moment, said Lord George, "500,000 able-bodied persons in Ireland living upon the funds of the state . . . commanded by a staff of 11,587 persons, employed upon works which have been variously described as 'works worse than idleness' . . . as 'public follies' and as 'works which will answer no other purpose than that of obstructing the public conveyances.' " Yet, as he pointed out, there were in Ireland only 123 miles of railway and 164 miles only under construction. He proposed that the destitute should be employed on a scheme which would be financed by Government loans up to £16,000,000, advanced at 3½ per

---

7. Reports Inspecting Officers, February 13, 1847, T 64/363 A. Captain Anderson to Routh, February 9, 1847, T 64/362 A. Captain Glascock to Trevelyan, February 20, 1847, Comm. Corr. II, p. 155. A. C. G. Bishop to Trevelyan, February 14, 1847, T 64/362 A.
8. Major Burns Report, February 6, 1847, T 64/363 A. Captain Kennedy Report, February 13, 1847, ibid. Captain Bull Report, February 20, 1847, ibid.

cent, the loan to be repaid with interest in 37 years, and the railways taken as security.

Trevelyan had already considered railway construction as a means of relief, and on October 6, 1846, in a long letter to Mr. Labouchere, he had pointed out the objections. The only item of railway construction requiring unskilled manual labour was earthworks, and that expenditure was only one-third of the whole. The most distressed of the population would not be reached, because railway lines were not constructed through impoverished districts, and far from giving employment to the helpless and destitute "the object of railway companies is to select the ablest labourers who will give the best return for their wages." Finally, railways were not permitted, under their Acts, to borrow until half the amount of their shares was paid up; as Irish railways were in a bad financial state, only two railways in Ireland would be eligible.[9]

Lord George Bentinck's Bill was defeated. But, later, Parliament voted a sum of £620,000 for loans to Irish railways which were able to establish that half their capital was paid up and were also able to spend a sum from their own resources equal to the loan. Only one line qualified, the South Western, running between Dublin and Cork, and railway construction therefore played a negligible part in relief during the famine.[10]

When about two weeks of the six allowed for the establishment of soup kitchens had passed, the Treasury sent a minute to the Board of Works, reminding them that the public works should be closed "as soon as the means of subsistence have been provided for the destitute in each neighbourhood"; to establish sufficient soup kitchens to feed the armies of the destitute had, however, proved impossible. By February 20, for instance, in Killarney there was only one soup kitchen for 10,000

---

9. Lord George Bentinck, H of C, February 4, 1847, Hansard, Vol. 89, pp. 773–804. B. Disraeli, *Lord George Bentinck: A Political Biography* (1852), p. 375. Trevelyan to Mr. Labouchere, October 6, 1846, B of W Corr. I, pp. 27, 28. Trevelyan to Col. Jones, April 8, 1847, T 64/363 B.

10. Trevelyan, *Crisis*, p. 133.

persons, and Tarbert had two "small establishments" for 18,000. The workhouses were full; on January 23 there were already 108,487 persons in institutions built to take 100,480;[11] and those who had no money, no employment, and no soup kitchen within reach, were doomed to starve.

In Leitrim there was a "fearful measure of distress," wrote Captain Layard, the Board of Works' Inspector. "Two cart loads of orphans, whose parents had died of starvation, were turned away from the workhouse yesterday." Something must be done; and he dashed off a list of suggestions. Why not a soup shop at every police barracks throughout the country? Why not the immediate establishment of a provision depot at Mohill? Why not put small stores of meal in schoolhouses, to be guarded by police or military? *"Something must be done,"* he repeated, urgently underlining his words, *"and that without delay."*[12]

Horrors were reported; at a farm in Caheragh, County Cork, a woman and her two children were found dead and half-eaten by dogs; in a neighbouring cottage five more corpses, which had been dead several days, were lying; and Father John O'Sullivan, parish priest of Kenmare, found "a room full of dead people"; a man, still living, was lying in bed with a dead wife and two dead children, while a starving cat was eating another dead infant.

Commander Caffyn, of H.M. Steam Sloop *Scourge*, "a man of undoubted honour and veracity," wrote a letter on February 15 which Trevelyan described as "awful." He had been discharging a cargo of meal for the Society of Friends at Skull, where a population of 18,000 inhabited a parish 21 miles in extent; and three-quarters of that population were skeletons, with swelling of the limbs and diarrhoea universal. In one cabin four adults and three children were crouched, silent, over a fire, while in another room a man and woman lay in bed, mere skeletons, the woman shrieking for food, the man past speech. The son of

---

11. Treasury Minute, February 16, 1847, Correspondence from January 1847–March 1847. Second part Board of Works Series, 1847 (797), LII, p. 155 (B of W Corr., II). Commander Stuart to Trevelyan, February 20, 1847, ibid., p. 210. Capt. Norris Report, February 20, 1847, T 64/363 A.

12. Captain Layard Report, February 14, 1847, Distress Papers 1473.

these people had been on the public works, and earned 8*d*. a day, which was not enough to keep the family from starvation, and he himself was now ill from hunger. These had been prosperous people.

In a second cabin a mother and daughter, reduced to skins stretched over bones, lay in bed. "Both must be dead by this time."

The third cabin contained an old woman and her daughter, whose husband had deserted her, with three little children. The grandmother had already died and was lying in the room, but her daughter was too exhausted to move her body.

The fourth cabin also contained a corpse which had been lying there for four days—no one could be found with sufficient strength to take it away.

Commander Caffyn saw a mass of bodies buried without coffins, "simply a few inches below the soil; when warm weather comes and they decompose there must be a pestilence." Bodies half-eaten by rats were an ordinary sight; "two dogs were shot while tearing a body to pieces." "Never in my life," wrote Commander Caffyn, "have I seen such wholesale misery."[13]

Numbers of landlords and middlemen now cleared subdivided estates of their swarming population. High rents had made subdivision tolerable, but this year rents had not been paid, and without the potato they would never be paid again. Wheat was to be substituted for the potato, and the minute holdings resulting from sub-division were a hopeless obstacle to wheat culture. "It is evident," wrote Mr. Todhunter, a member of the Central Relief Committee of the Society of Friends on January 23, "that some landlords, forgetful of the claims of humanity and regardless of the Public Welfare, are availing themselves of the present calamity to effect a wholesale clearance of their estates."

All the same, the Government was determined to bring the

13. Bishop to Routh, February 19, 1847, Comm. Corr. II, p. 164. The Rev. J. O. O'Sullivan to Trevelyan, February 1847, T64/362A. Trevelyan to Sir John Burgoyne, February 18, 1847, Comm. Corr. II, pp. 160, 161. Commander Caffyn to Captain Hamilton, February 15, 1847, Comm. Corr. II, pp. 162–4.

public works to an end, and on February 22 the Board of Works sent out a circular to all inspecting officers instructing them to strike every possible name from the lists, as "the Public Works are drawing to a close."[14]

Inspecting officers, however, were powerless; the vast crowds of wretched, starving, and, in the Government's own phrase, "half-dying" wretches were beyond control. A hundred names might be struck off in a week, wrote Captain Kennedy, Inspector for Meath, but 150 new names come on every day. In Galway "lists after lists" were pouring into the Board of Works' Inspector's office, "containing hundreds of names representing people stated to be literally starving." Meanwhile, the relief committees had "almost ceased to act." In some places a committee of hopelessly unsuitable persons had been sanctioned; in Glenties, County Donegal, the chairman was a "tinker," as the gipsies of the Irish countryside were called, and two of the Guardians had got tickets for the public works; in others, committees refused to take the risk of discharging starving, desperate men. In Carlow the Inspecting Officer had to give the order to turn off 140 men himself, and in public, because the relief committee "could not be got to do it."[15]

---

14. Mr. Pim to Sir Robert Peel, January 23, 1847, Comm. Corr. II, p. 86. Circular No. 66, To Inspecting Officers from J. Walker, Secy. Office of Public Works, February 22, 1847, B of W Corr. II, p. 232.

15. Capt. Kennedy Report, February 13, 1847, T 64/363 A. Major Burns Report, January 16, 1847, B of W Corr. II, p. 127. Major Burns Report, January 23, 1847, ibid., p. 128. Lieut. Milward Report, February 6, 1847, T 64/363 A. Lieut. Hotham Report, February 20, 1847, ibid.

Peasant Diet in Eighteenth-Century Gévaudan

R.-J. BERNARD

How did our ancestors eat? What bearing did their diet have on their life expectancy? These questions are rightly on the minds of historians as they endeavor to understand the daily life of individuals and groups over the centuries in its most concrete aspects; but only too often the answers are difficult to find. As a tool to this end, more use could certainly be made of the "teeming wealth"[1] of the notarial archives, especially in regions of written law, where notaries' offices existed even in the most remote hamlets. In these areas, notaries played a much greater role in the major and minor affairs of everyone's life than in regions of customary law, since even the payment of a very small sum was notarized. This is what I shall try to show on the basis of the minutes of the office of *maître* Antoine Bonnet,[2] royal notary in the town of Châteauneuf-de-Randon in the Gévaudan between 1754 and 1788. Presently the *chef-lieu* of a

SOURCE: "L'alimentation paysanne en Gévaudan au XVIIIe siècle" by R.-J. Bernard, in *Annales: Économies, Sociétés, Civilisations*, no. 6 (November–December, 1969), pp. 1449–1467. Reprinted by permission of *Annales*.

1. The expression is Pierre Goubert's, who took chronological samples of this source in his thesis on Beauvais and the Beauvaisis, 1600–1730.
2. Archives Départmentales; hereafter cited as A.D., Lozère; III–E 5802–5834. I am preparing a thesis on life in the Gévaudan from the seventeenth to the twentieth century under the direction of Pierre Vilar.

canton in the department of Lozère and renowned since the middle of the sixteenth century for its cattle and sheep markets, the influence of the town extended (and continues to extend)[3] over the southern extremity of the Margeride, the plateaux of the Gévaudan between the Margeride and the valley of the Allier, the compact mass of the forest of Mercoire and the little Causse de Montbel, better known as the plain of Montbel, even though it is situated at an altitude of between 1,100 and 1,250 meters.

Since the old French law was much more concerned with the family and the community than is the civil code, the obligation to provide food for aged parents or grandparents, children, or close relatives temporarily or permanently unable to provide for their own needs was very firmly stated and carefully worked out as to its implementation. This was true in the customary as well as in the written law. Thus it is not surprising that a certain number of wills and marriage contracts included food pensions, that is, a fixed, unchangeable quantity of various foodstuffs[4] to be given every year, in one or more installments, to the person designated by name in the document. In the wills, the pension was established in favor of the wife, in case the husband should die first; in the marriage contracts, it was established in favor of the father or mother of one of the future spouses. In most cases,

---

3. This is shown by the addresses of the notary's clients. A cartographic representation of the addresses of the clientele of notaries' offices would seem to be a very exact way of measuring the impact of *bourgs* and small towns on the surrounding countryside and to establish areas of influence that would be much more valuable for the analysis of local social and economic configurations than official administrative and fiscal boundaries. This suggestion applies mainly to regions of written law.

4. Sometimes the food pension in kind is replaced by a lifetime annuity in money, regardless of the fortune of the parties to the contract. Thus on April 2, 1761, Jean Granier, of the parish of Arsenc-de-Randon, reserves for himself a lifetime annuity of 24 livres in the marriage contract of his daughter Claudine; on August 31, 1763, Anne Marie de Fage, widow of Jean Rozier, advocate at the *parlement*, stipulates a lifetime annuity of 600 livres for herself in the contract of marriage between her son George Rozier, president of the *Bureau de l'élection* of Hautu Rouerg, *conseiller du Roy*, and mayor of Millau, and Marie de Lahondes de Laborie, daughter of the *conseiller du Roy* and mayor of Châteauneuf-de-Randon; on February 23, 1764, Marie Bohomme, widow of Jean Peytavin, is given a sum of 700 livres for her personal needs in the marriage contract of her son Michel, *laboureur* at Chadenet.

one of the future spouses, or even both, had lost one parent[5] and the survivor wanted to assure his or her livelihood in case of a rift with the young couple. This was a necessary precaution, since the fact that the "old folks" and the "young folks" lived together under the same roof provided ample fuel for quarrels, especially when matters of self-interest were added to the conflict of personalities and generations. It must be added that until very recently this cohabitation has stifled the initiative of the more open of the young peasants and thus perpetuated a most regrettable stagnation in the agriculture of the Lozère. Nor was the practice of the right of the eldest helpful; quite to the contrary. If the eldest son inherited the land and the farming tools, he had to pay his younger brothers and sisters their portion (*légitime*), the share of the paternal and maternal inheritance to which they were legally entitled, which represented a heavy burden.[6] There was a strong temptation to cut corners when it came to taking care of an old mother or father, a crippled or retarded brother or sister; and a new son-in-law or daughter-in-law was very apt to reinforce this tendency. Therefore, the head of the family in his will or the surviving parent at the occasion of the marriage of the eldest son or daughter who was to take over the *"oustal"* (the family homestead), ensured their future by stipulating a food pension for themselves or by constituting a *rente* in favor of a permanently disabled child. I have found some thirty documents of this kind in the minutes of the office of Antoine Bonnet for the period 1754–67, to which I am limiting my preliminary investigation.

5. Does this mean that the ages at marriage were rather advanced? This is a difficult problem of demography, for in many parish registers the ages of the future spouses are not stated. They could be established by finding the dates of birth, but that is not always possible if one of the partners comes from another parish; furthermore, in the parishes we are studying (northeast Gévaudan), the existing birth records are quite spotty from the end of the seventeenth to the beginning of the eighteenth century.

6. Here again, the testimony of the notarial minutes is eloquent. To take only those of Antoine Bonnet, fully two-thirds of the obligations (statements of debts, receipts, *précaires, antichrèses,* and other disguised forms of mortgages) were contracted in order to pay the portions, which were often stretched out over an entire lifetime or even passed on to the next generation.

Years	Wills		Marriage Contracts	
	Total number	With a food pension	Total number	With a food pension
1754–1756	7	—	16	3
1757–1759	13	2	22	—
1759–1760	10	—	13	3
1760–1762	12	2	18	5
1762–1763	12	—	10	—
1763–1764	13	2	14	4
1764–1766	30	2	19	4
1766–1767	23	—	7	—
Total	120	8	119	19

This, then, is a small but perfectly valid sample, for in the region of written law where the *senatus consultum velleianum* was invoked to protect the wife's dotal property from squandering or mismanagement by the husband practically everyone used a notary, even the very poor. There were a great many wills and marriage contracts in which stereotyped and high-sounding legal language was quite incapable of disguising the poverty of the contracting parties. There was, for instance, the case of the future spouses who "constitute each other's goods as common property," with the bride giving her future husband "full power of attorney," but in which the goods brought into the marriage by either bride or groom were not enumerated—and that for very good reasons. Or the heads of families richer in progeny than in hard cash who in their wills bequeathed to each of their children "the legitimate portion to which they are entitled" without going into any further details. Many more such examples could be cited.

I have brought together the results of my research in three large tables that require some explanation. Table 1 gives the composition, in local measurement, of the various food rations stipulated in each one of these pensions, and a note indicates how these measurements were converted into modern units.

The products mentioned here were widely used[7] (and continued to be widely used up to the time when food habits changed in the wake of the general rise in the standard of living of the rural population over the last fifty years, and particularly since World War II). Thus, they give an accurate idea of the peasant diet in the second half of the eighteenth century.

Cereals formed the basis of that diet: rye, the most suitable cereal for making bread, and barley. In bread making, rye flour was quite often "stretched" with barley flour (nine out of twenty-seven pensions), this being an indication of the low standard of living of the peasants of the Gévaudan at that time; for by the middle of the nineteenth century, barley was no longer considered suitable for bread making and was used exclusively for animal feed. A small proportion of the barley harvest was made into "pearled" or "cleaned" barley by a special process in a special kind of mill, and the end product was somewhat similar to rice.[8] Simmered with a small piece of salt pork for three or four hours, it yielded a tasty and refreshing soup, greatly appreciated by the harvest hands for their noonday meal. As the stocks of "pearled" barley had to be carefully husbanded, this soup appeared on the menu only in summer, during the harvest, or else at the occasion of some family celebration. Wheat appears only once in our table, namely, in the parish of Allenc, which is situated on the Causse de Montbel, where good wheat land is found; and even there it represents

---

7. It should be indicated here that the peasant diet in the Gévaudan was considerably improved by the introduction of the potato, which gradually began to be grown from 1815 on, not without encountering a great deal of resistance. In the Velay region, the potato appears in this very type of document at the same time and even somewhat earlier.

8. In a *Mémoire sur le département de Lozère*, preserved at the Military Archives at Vincennes (M.R. 1274) and most probably dating from the years 1836–40, the staff lieutenant de Caulaincourt writes that the peasants of Lozère live on rye bread, milk products, pork, potatoes, chestnuts (in the Cevennes), turnips, kitchen vegetables, and rice. This is certainly a misunderstanding: the officer, whose knowledge of the Lozère seems superficial, must have taken pearled barley for rice. To this day, pearled barley is much appreciated, but it can be bought ready-made at the grocery store.

Table 1
ANNUAL FOOD RATIONS
(Converted into Liters for Grains and Kilograms for Other Products)

Origin of the pension and the local measure used	Rye	Barley	Wheat	Chestnuts	Cabbage, turnips, garden herbs	Salt lard	Cheese	Butter
1. P,M (MCH)	5 cartalières (65.20 l.)	5 cartalières (65.20 l.)			1 sack turnips			4 livres (1.743 kg.)
2. P,M (MV)	8 cartes (120 l.)			6 cartes (90 l.)				
3. P,M (MCH)	5 cartalières (65.20 l.)	5 cartalières (65.20 l.)						
4. C,M (MB)	6 cartes (121.08 l.)	6 cartes (121.08 l.)	3 cartes (60.54 l.)		Needs of cabbage and turnips	10 livres (4.358 kg.)	5 livres (2.179 kg.)	5 livres (2.179 kg.)
5. C,M (MCH)	25 cartalières (316 l.)				Needs of cabbage and turnips	15 livres (6.537 kg.)	15 livres (6.537 kg.)	10 livres (4.358 kg.)
6. ½C,M (MCH)	18 cartalières (227.52 l.)	7 cartalières (89.58 l.)			Needs of cabbage and turnips		5 livres (2.179 kg.)	5 livres (2.179 kg.)
7. ½C,M (MCH)	16 cartalières (202.24 l.)				Needs of turnips and garden prod.		6 livres (2.614 kg.)	6 livres (2.614 kg.)

8. P,M (MCH)	3 cartes (186.60 l.)						
9. C,M (MCH)	35 cartalières (422.40 l.)			30 livres (13.074 kg.)	12 livres 1/2 (5.447 kg.)	12 livres 1/2 (5.447 kg.)	
10. P,M (MCH)	10 cartalières (126.40 l.)						
11. C,M (MM)	12 cartes (180 l.)	4 cartes (60 l.)	Needs of cabbage and turnips	8 livres (3.486 kg.)	6 livres (2.614 kg.)	6 livres (2.614 kg.)	
12. C,M (MB)	8 cartes (161.44 l.)	4 cartes (80.72 l.)	Needs of cabbage and turnips	6 livres (2.614 kg.)	6 livres (2.614 kg.)	6 livres (2.614 kg.)	
13. C,M (ML)	6 cartes (357.60 l.)		"Small needs" of cabbage and turnips	20 livres (8.716 kg.)	12 livres (5.228 kg.)	7 livres (3.268 kg.)	
14. C,T (MCH)	32 cartalières (404.48 l.)		Needs of cabbage and turnips	12 livres (5.228 kg.)	6 livres (2.614 kg.)	6 livres (2.614 kg.)	

Table 1 (continued)
ANNUAL FOOD RATIONS
(Converted into Liters for Grains and Kilograms for Other Products)

Origin of the pension and the local measure used	Rye	Barley	Wheat	Chestnuts	Cabbage, turnips, garden herbs	Salt lard	Cheese	Butter
15. C,T (ML)	8 cartes (476.60 l.)				Needs of cabbage and garden prod.:1 cart of turnips	20 livres (8.716 kg.)	20 livres (8.716 kg.)	20 livres (8.716 kg.)
16. C,T (ML)	6 cartes (357.60 l.)	1 carte (59.60 l.)			Needs of cabbage, turnips	20 livres (8.716 kg.)	6 livres (2.614 kg.)	10 livres (4.358 kg.)
17. C,T (MCH)	6 cartes (370.20 l.)	3 cartes (178.80 l.)			Needs of cabbage, turnips	15 livres (6.537 kg.)	12 livres (5.229 kg.)	10 livres (4.358 kg.)
18. C,T (MCH)	20 cartalières (252.80 l.)	12 cartalières (151.68 l.)				15 livres (6.537 kg.)	7 livres 1/2 (3.268 kg.)	7 livres 1/2 (3.268 kg.)
19. P,T (MCH)	36 cartalières (455.04 l.)							
20. P,T (ML)	1 carte (59.60 l.)							

21. *P, T* (ML)	10 carta-lières (119.20 l.)			
22. *P, T* (MCH) (in 1616)	3 setiers (358.59 l.)			
23. *C, T* (MCH) (in 1615)	7 cartes (443.40 l.)		1 car-tay Ron	1 car-tay Ron	5 livres (2.179 kg.)

NOTE: This table has been established in the following manner:
M = Contract of marriage (notarized documents from which I have extracted the food pensions on which the present article is based)
T = Will or testament (notarized documents from which I have extracted the food pensions on which the present article is based)
As a convenience, every pension has been assigned a number in boldface.
As everywhere in France, the local measures for weights and capacity were extremely complex, since they varied from town to town (as Voltaire said: "We change measures as we change post-horses").
For the conversions into modern measures, I have used:
1. An exhaustive study by M. Albert Fayet, a judge in the arrondissement of Orange, published in 1885 in the *Bulletin de la Société d'Agriculture, des Sciences et Lettres de la Lozère*, "Usages et réglements locaux ayant force de loi dans le département de la Lozère et recueillies avec l'aide de MM. les juges de paix de ce département." This title suggests that the memory of the old measures was still very lively at the end of the nineteenth century.
2. "Table des comparaisons entre anciens poids et mesures de la Lozère et le nouveau système métrique," based on the method of conversion of the avoué Cornut (Year II of the Republic). Cf. *Bulletin de la Société d'Agriculture, des Sciences, Lettres et Arts de la Lozère,* 1899.
3. "Notes et documents sur les anciennes mesures de grains en Gévaudan" by Charles Porée, archivist of the department of Lozère. Published in the collective volume *Le moyen âge* (Paris, 1901). Cf. also A. D. Lozère 80–H–70.
Local measures mentioned in the Table: MCH = measure of Châteauneuf-de-Randon; MV = measure of Villefort; MB = measure of Bleymard; MM = measure of Mende; ML = measure of Langogne. The *carte,* the principal measure of capacity for grain, held more at Châteauneuf-de-Randon than at Langogne. No wonder that seigneurial proprietors were so careful to spell out the measures in which dues in kind were to be paid in their *Terriers* and *Livres de reconnaissances.* . . .

only 20 percent of the cereal used for bread, as against 40 percent rye and 40 percent barley. The only and exceptional ration of chestnuts is found at Prevenchères, in the chestnut forest of the Cévennes.

Many of these food pensions included vegetables in the form of cabbage and turnips. Only two cases stipulate very approximate quantities (nos. 1 and 5), namely, one sack and one cart; otherwise, the beneficiary of the pension was guaranteed only his "needs" or even his "small needs": in other words, he could take from the vegetable patch adjoining the house as many cabbages and turnips as he needed, so long as the "young folks," especially the son-in-law or the daughter-in-law, were not too stingy. It all depended on how the family got along. . . .

What was meant by "garden needs" (no. 7) or "soup vegetables" (no. 15)? This is rather difficult to establish with any precision.[9] No doubt, these needs included dandelions and a few salads, the only vegetables eaten raw in those days, and that in small quantities, but apparently enough to make up, in part at least, for the deficiencies in beriberi- and scurvy-preventing vitamins of the diet. To this we must add onions, quite small by comparison to the onions we know today, celery, and carrots, all of which were used to flavor the usual soup made of cabbage, turnips, bread, and a small piece of lard.

Animal products are represented only by salt pork, which was extremely fat and had almost no lean meat under a very thick rind.[10] We therefore classify it under fats in the dietary balance sheet of these rations. One is surprised to find neither ham nor

9. In view of the very slow modernization of the Gévaudan, I have frequently complemented my information by availing myself of oral traditions—in other words, by interviewing old persons (over seventy) including an uncle almost one hundred years old and my mother. The latter told me, among other things, that around 1900 in my maternal grandfather's family (nine children), one liter of oil lasted several months, since salad appeared on the family table only very rarely, in the summer and fall. Otherwise, raw vegetables, such as the uncooked carrots we eat today, were totally unknown. Aside from the potato, diet and food habits had not changed very much since the second half of the eighteenth century.

10. These rinds were collected in an earthen jar, and when they were quite rancid they served to flavor the cabbage soup.

sausage nor any other kind of prepared pork products (*charcuterie*) in these pensions, but the fact can easily be explained. Even though exact data are not available, it is quite clear that the pigs of that time were very poorly nourished and yielded neither the weight nor the quantity of meat of today's pigs,[11] which are fattened with bran, processed grain, potatoes, and whey, the residue in *tome* (cheese) and butter making. This was not always the case. At the beginning of this century, not to go back any further, pigs that were being fattened hardly ever tasted grain or bran—food for people came first. As for the by-products of cheese and butter making, they were consumed by humans. The *rebarbe* was a most welcome addition to an otherwise rather meager meal, especially in poor families; it was obtained by mixing whey and the residue from making the *tome* in an earthenware vessel called a *"terrou"* [hereafter, italicized words enclosed in quotation marks refer to local dialect]. Sometimes the *rebarbe* was made to ferment by placing the *terrou* under a haystack, and this process yielded a kind of runny and very strong-smelling cheese of which some peasants, including my maternal grandfather, were very fond, and which was somewhat similar to the *cancailotte* of Franche Comté.

The *tome* was the typical cheese of the Lozère and remains so in the places where it is still produced. It is very different from what is called *tome* in Savoy: that of Lozère is a firm cheese whose color changes from yellow-white to very deep ivory marbled with red or green during the aging process; in time the originally thin crust becomes hard and thick, and after it has

11. This was bound to affect the production of prepared pork products; on the other hand, we must also take into account the feasts connected with the slaughtering and preparation of the family pig. Furthermore, just as for the "needs" of cabbage, turnips, and soup vegetables, there were certain customs and realities of day-to-day living: unless they were excessively stingy or fundamentally hostile, the "young folks" would certainly not deny their old father or mother a bit of sausage and a slice of ham or exclude them from the feast when the pig was killed.

Here again, it all depended on the harmony (or lack thereof) among the members of the family; and all too often the beneficiary of a food pension was reduced to begging for favors. These patriarchal families of the Gévaudan did not always present an idyllic and edifying picture.

been kept for four to six months in a cool and humid place, usually the *"patouille"* or *"souillarde"* (a back kitchen connected with the stable), it shows mold similar to that of Roquefort or *fourme d'Ambert*. At that point the *tome* becomes a fermented cheese; but it was usually consumed before it reached this stage.

The peasant diet as we see it through these food pensions was thus based on cereals, consumed mainly in the form of bread. This bread was eaten in various ways: with a piece of lard or some *tome* on ordinary days; with a little ham or sausage on Sundays or feast days, although this would suppose a well-stocked larder *("charnier")*;[12] rubbed with an onion, spread with *rebarbe*, or soaked in soup, which it served to thicken.

In order to appraise the nutritional value of this diet and to show its deficiencies, we should know the quality of the products consumed and compare them with present-day farm products. Over the last ten years, a few farmers have begun to use various kinds of flour, feed cakes, enriched products, and molasses to improve the feed of their livestock; they have also begun to spread chemical fertilizer on their fields and to regenerate their hayfields, even to replace them with artificial meadows. But in the northeast of the Gévaudan, this evolution is only just beginning, so that we can perfectly well make use of oral traditions, even my own childhood memories going back to the years immediately before World War II, when the old ways of the Lozère were still very much alive.

The bread was kneaded at the farm[13] and baked in the communal oven of the village (only the *mas* and very large farms had their own oven). Its preparation mobilized the energies of everyone in the house every other week in the summer and once a month in the winter (less bread was eaten in winter, especially if it was stale). The finished product took the form of

---

12. The *charnier* was a cool, dry place protected from rats and other undesirable creatures, where butter, flour, salted meats, and possibly the stock of wine were kept. It was often located close to the master bedroom.

13. The kneading trough (or *maits à paitrir*) was an essential piece of equipment in the peasant household, as we can see in inventories after death and evaluations of the partners' dotal property in marriage contracts.

large round loaves weighing 5–8 kg. Its black crust was so thick that the head of the family needed a very sharp knife to cut off slices for the rest of the family;[14] the heavy and compact inside of the bread was light brown, and the paste it formed when mixed with saliva stuck to the roof of the mouth before it was swallowed. These characteristics were due to the very coarse grinding of the grains between the roughly cut and uneven stones of the water mills (sometimes the flour contained grains that were not ground at all, just barely crushed) with a very heavy level of bolting (90 percent),[15] so that most of the bran was left in the flour. This yielded a bread as nutritious and rich in vitamins as today's so-called "whole grain" breads; it was about as digestible as the more or less adulterated white breads modern city-dwellers can buy, and it tasted rather good. After all, rye bread is again becoming fashionable today, especially for eating with oysters. Finally, its high roughage content favored intestinal activity. I sometimes nostalgically evoke memories of carefree childhood vacations: the paterfamilias (my uncle) cutting the loaf of bread amid the deferential silence of his family, having first traced the sign of the cross on its crust with the tip of his knife in order to call the blessing of heaven down upon this earthly food that man's hard labor had wrenched from a naturally barren soil.

The other foodstuffs fully deserved to be called "natural products," since nothing artificial was used to produce them. They did not contain any substance harmful to the organism, but the way they were served and preserved was perhaps not as good as that of present-day products. Thus the quality and preservation of butter and *tome* depended (and continue to depend) on the sanitary condition and the feeding of the cows. At the end of winter and in early spring, when the indoor period is coming to an end and when the hay, even generously mixed with straw, is almost gone, the cows are fed smaller and smaller rations (espe-

---

14. He alone had this right, and no one would have dreamed of infringing upon it. Only the men ate at the table; the women served them and then ate their meal in silence by the hearth.
15. Cf. the note attached to Table 2.

cially in the old days), and the production of milk diminishes accordingly. Furthermore, the peasants think that the quality of the butter and the *tome* is rather mediocre at this time of the year: a great many *tomes* become mildewed and infected with maggots (in the old days they were eaten anyway, maggots and all), a great many cakes of butter become rancid right away. . . . By contrast, in early summer and at the time of the second mowing, when the grass is thick and green, the butter and the *tome* acquire a flavor that is the delight of the connoisseur; and they also keep very well. The quality of the grass and the pastures is important. . . . The care with which these products are prepared influences their quality as well: butter made from cream that is not completely separated from the whey, not sufficiently kneaded, or handled by a careless or unclean farmer's wife will not keep and soon becomes rancid. I myself have sometimes found in one of these cakes of butter of doubtful quality, between some drops of whey, one or two long curly hairs that the farmer's wife had been negligent enough to drop while beating her churn.

In the Gévaudan, all the pork products were (and are) preserved by salting. Pepper[16] is added to season ham and sausage. However, it was important to add a sufficient quantity of salt, so that proper salting depended on the price of salt. If it was too expensive, the poorest peasants did not add enough salt to their meat and then the lard soon became rancid and worms attacked the sausages. This was one of the many compelling reasons for hating the *gabelle* (salt tax) and for vilifying the *gabelous* who were not above raising the price of salt illegally and cheating on its quality.[17]

---

16. This practice was already established in the eighteenth century: a number of village communities that rented their outlying mountain meadows and pastures *(herbes champêtres)* to the owners of migrating herds of sheep from Lower Languedoc stipulated in their rent contracts that the *baile* (the manager and head shepherd) who brought the herds was to furnish a certain amount of pepper.

17. For all this, I refer the reader to an article, "Note sur le prix du sel en Gévaudan au XVIIIe siècle," I wrote for the May–June issue of *Lou Pais*, a delightful little local review published monthly in Montpellier.

Table 2 gives the daily rations in grams, on the basis of which I have divided the food pensions into three categories:

Table 2
DAILY RATIONS
(in Grams)

Pension	Bread			Butter	Cheese	Salt lard
	Annual cereal ration (in kg.)	Daily ration	Equivalent of bread			
1. P	100.30	270.47	243.42	4.77		
2. P	161.70	443.00	398.70			
3. P	100.30	270.47	243.42			
4. C	233.07	638.00	574.20	5.88	5.88	11.93
5. C	243.32	666.60	600.00	11.93	17.90	17.90
6. 1/2 C	244.16	668.80	601.90	5.88	5.88	
7. 1/2 C	155.72	426.60	383.94	7.05	7.05	
8. P	146.00	400.00	360.00			
9. C	340.64	933.26	840.00	14.70	14.90	35.80
10. P	97.32	240.00				
11. C	184.80	506.30	455.67	7.05	7.05	9.55
12. C	186.46	510.83	459.75	7.05	7.05	7.05
13. C	275.35	754.30	678.87	8.95	14.30	23.87
14. C	311.44	853.26	768.00	7.05	7.05	14.32
15. C	345.13	945.56	851.00	23.87	24.36	23.87
16. C	321.24	880.10	792.09	11.93	7.05	23.87
17. C	429.66	1,177.15	1,059.43	11.93	14.10	17.90
18. C	311.44	853.26	767.93	8.95	8.95	17.90
19. P	350.38	959.90	863.91			
20. P	45.89	125.80	113.22			
21. P	91.78	251.60	226.44			
22. P	276.03	838.40	754.56			
23. C	341.41	935.10	841.60	5.88	?	?

NOTE: The weight of the annual ration of cereal was arrived at by assuming that rye and barley have the same average density of 0.77 as wheat, which was indicated by Georges and Genèvieve Frèche on page 13 of their book *Prix du pain, du vin et des légumes à Toulouse, de 1486 à 1868* (Paris: P.U.F., 1967). In the absence of more specific information, I have adopted this approximation, which, however, should not unduly falsify my calculations.

The equivalent in bread of the daily cereal ration has been calculated on the basis of a level of bolting of 90 percent, which seems very high when we compare it to the present-day legal level (between 72 and 80 percent) practiced by the bakeries. However, this level of 90 percent was habitual in the Gévaudan as long as the peasants baked their own bread. This was confirmed by some old people I was able to question on the subject. Finally, recall that in 1943 the level of bolting was raised to 89 percent.... Moreover, in case of food shortage or poverty, this level must certainly have been close to 100 percent, not to forget the practice of sometimes adding rather unusual substances in order to stretch the flour.

Complete pensions (C), which provided for giving cereals, salt lard, butter, cheese, and "needs" of cabbage, turnips, and soup vegetables.

Partial pensions (P), cereals only, except for no. 1, which specified an insignificant amount of butter as a supplement.

Semicomplete pensions (½ C), with cereals, the "needs" of cabbage, turnips, "soup vegetables," cheese, and butter, but without salt lard.

The partial and semicomplete pensions (eleven in all) usually specified rather small daily rations of bread; only three of them (nos. 6, 19, 22) assured their recipients of more than 500 g. of bread per day. Perhaps these persons had some resources of their own, such as a small, patiently accumulated amount of cash; or else they were also helped by their other children.

If the twelve complete pensions provided for a reasonable daily quantity of bread, i.e., at least 500 g. (except for nos. 11 and 12), the rations of butter, lard, and cheese were very modest indeed. Tables 1 and 2 indicate that the annual rations varied between a minimum of 1.743 kg. (pension no. 1, which, however, belongs to the partial category) and a maximum of 8.716 kg. These quantities amount to a daily average which is higher than 20 g. in only four cases (nos. 9, 13, 15, 16), including case no. 9, providing the almost Rabelaisian largess of 35.80 g. of lard per day. . . .

These small amounts are not surprising in view of the state of traditional agriculture in the Gévaudan,[18] where livestock and

18. On this point, see my article "Les nuits de fumade d'aprés le compoix et cadastre de Belvezet en 1630," *Revue du Gévaudan, des Causses et des Cévennes*, 1965. Furthermore, I have found in the *Terriers* and *Livres de Reconnaissances* of the parishes and seigneuries of the northeast Gévaudan (the subject of my thesis) only a few very exceptional cases of dues to be paid in butter and cheese, further proof that these products were scarce. Similarly, the only poultry products appearing as dues are chickens; and they are mentioned in the curious form of ½ chicken, ⅓ or ¼ chicken—i.e., one chicken every two, three, or four years; or else ¾ or 2 and ⅓ [sic] chickens—i.e., three chickens every four years or two chickens every three years. As for eggs, they never appear at all. It should be added that the price statistics (*mercuriales*) of the region (Langogne, Châteauneuf-de-Randon, abbey of Chambons) never included poultry products. This would indicate that they were very rare, so that there is no need to include poultry products in our study of peasant diet in the eighteenth century.

poultry played only a very minor role and where the milk production of the Aubrac cattle was very poor.[19]

Cheese, butter, and lard, then, appeared in very small amounts in these pensions; there was just enough of these to "make the bread," mainstay of the peasant diet, "go down."

The nutritional balance sheet[20] given in Table 3 corroborates these quantitative data.

The conclusion is inescapable that of the twelve complete pensions only two provided for more than the 2,400 calories needed for moderate work (nos. 15, 17), that only one (no. 19) comes close to this minimum, that *none* provided as much as 3,000 calories, and that three of them (nos. 4, 11, 12) yielded less than the 1,500 calories needed to sustain life. As for the partial and semicomplete pensions, six of them did not yield even 1,000 calories; one can only hope that they were complemented from other sources; otherwise, physiological damage and death were sure to ensue in very short order. These deficiencies and their consequences can be appreciated by recalling the tragic memories of the Nazi occupation.[21]

It might be objected that these insufficient rations were destined for the aged, who were less active and had smaller food requirements. This argument does not stand up to a critical examination. First of all, what was meant in the eighteenth century, and in the the Gévaudan, by "aged persons"? The demographic studies I am pursuing in the context of my thesis[22] show

19. On the eve of World War II, the average milk production of this breed was 3 to 10 liters per day, depending on the age and health of the animals and the feed they received. There does not seem to have been any progress since the last years of the nineteenth century, and even much earlier. . . .

20. It was established on the basis of the excellent little book by Raymond Lalanne, *L'alimentation humaine*, 8th ed., Collection "Que sais-je?" (Paris: P.U.F., 1967).

21. Cf. M. Amouroux, *La vie quotidienne des Français sous l'occupation* (Paris: Fayard, 1966).

22. They concern the parishes of Allenc, Chasseradès, Luc, Arsenc-de-Randon, Saint-Jean-la-Foulhouze, and Chaudeyrac within their eighteenth-century limits, which do not necessarily coincide with the present-day communities, since a certain number of parishes were considered too large and consequently divided up in the middle of the nineteenth century. These are the only ones where fairly complete parish registers can be found and used quantitatively.

that life expectancy was about forty years, and that adult deaths occurred with great frequency between the ages of forty and fifty and, to a lesser degree, between the ages of fifty and sixty; in other words, at an age that can hardly be qualified as senility. The small number of solidly built people who lived on beyond the age of sixty should not mislead us.

Were the beneficiaries of these pensions "retired" in the modern sense of the word? Certainly not. The peasant worked, and had to work, up to the time of death. His family did not hesitate to remind him of this fact, sometimes quite directly. The harsh country with its rude climate and barren soil; the ambiance of hopeless poverty permeating everyday life; families who were often much more prolific than they could afford to be and who, because of ignorance and religious fervor, remained untouched by the "dread secrets" of birth control—widely known and used though these were in other regions; a very strong acquisitiveness, exacerbated by constant shortness, but probably inherent in the peasant mentality[23] and consciousness—all these things made the existence of idlers and useless mouths intolerable. Wills and marriage contracts very often contained clauses stipulating that old parents, old uncles, younger brothers and sisters fed and housed by the eldest son in the family homestead until their majority (fixed at the age of twenty-five at that time) were under the firm obligation of working "to the best of their ability" for the "prosperity of the family" and "for the interest of the designated heir." These are literal quotations of the set formulations employed. One has to have lived in this kind of rural

---

23. Even though the study of peasant mentality and consciousness has been somewhat neglected by the specialists of rural history, this acquisitiveness was seen both by P. de Saint-Jacob *(Les paysans de la Bourgogne du Nord)* and by P. Bois *(Les paysans de l'Ouest)*. In his recently published thesis, Abel Poitrineau shows very well how the extreme poverty of the peasants of Haute-Auvergne—hardly better off than those of the Gévaudan—made them even more interested in money and hoarding cash. Many more examples could be taken from literary works about life in the countryside: while Émile Zola's *La terre* is perhaps overly intellectualized and marked by Parisian standards, several short stories by Guy de Maupassant immediately come to mind, as well as two admirable peasant novels, *Jacquou le Croquant* by Eugène le Roy and *La vie d'un simple* by Emile Guillaumin.

environment to realize how strongly the iron law of work to the point of exhaustion ("you shall work until you have one foot in the grave") pervaded the peasant mentality, exposing those who could not—or could no longer—work to a treatment that was not always compatible with the outward marks of respect shown to the aged or with the requirements of Christian charity.

Not only were these rations insufficient in calories; the imbalances and deficiencies in their composition and quantity further compromised the already limited use the body could make of them. According to the modern tenets of nutrition, the daily food intake must furnish a certain number of energy-producing substances—namely, protids, lipids, and glucides. What was the situation here?

1. Proteins are the only source of nitrogens and the life-giving amino acids. It is necessary to consume at the very least 1 g. of these per kg. of body weight. Let us take a look at Table 3. Considering only the complete and semicomplete pensions, we note that six of them furnish less than 50 g. of protids, clearly not enough for a grown person's work. One of them (no. 17) furnishes somewhat more, namely, 88.69 g. and only seven seem to be satisfactory, furnishing between 50 and 75 g., which would be the proper amount for the normal adult body weight (nos. 5, 9, 13, 14, 15, 16, 18). Clearly, there is a lack of balance in these rations. . . . To be fully effective, 40 percent of the protein intake should be of animal origin, for protids of animal origin are much higher in amino acids than those of plant origin. This is not the case here: the only animal proteins we find come from cheese, and they amount to no more than 2 to 5 percent of the total. How could it be otherwise, when meat, the prime source of animal proteins, was practically absent from this diet, the very rare occasions when salted pork products were consumed not withstanding. There was, then, a shortage of animal proteins that hampered the growth of the child and jeopardized the health of the adult.

2. Lipids, or fats, furnish fatty acids, which are as indispensable to the support of life as the amino acids, since they keep up the body temperature. The daily minimum for adults is 40 g.; yet of the twelve complete pensions in Table 3 only three (nos. 9, 15, 17) furnish this minimum, despite the rather optimistic level we are postulating here, and one comes close to it (no. 16). This insufficiency was very

Table 3
NUTRITIONAL BALANCE SHEET OF THE RATIONS

Rations	Proteins (g.)			Lipids (g.)					Glucides (g.)			Trace Elements (mg.)			Calories	
	Bread	Cheese	Total	Bread	Butter	Cheese	Salt Lard	Total	Bread	Cheese	Total	Phosphorus	Calcium	Iron	Total	% from Bread
1. P	19.47			2.43				6.48	121.71			487.90	234.25	8.13	603.24	94.86
2. P	31.85			3.98	4.05				195.70			717.66	239.20	11.96	919.90	100
3. P	19.47			2.43					121.71			487.90	234.25	8.13	472.26	100
4. C	45.93	1.64	47.57	5.74	4.99	1.76	10.14	22.63	287.01	0.02	287.03	1,070.62	386.26	17.26	1,576.07	89.80
5. C	48.00	5.01	53.01	6.00	10.14	5.37	15.21	36.72	300.00	0.71	300.71	1,171.28	486.49	18.10	1,665.51	83.20
6. 1/2 C	48.03	1.64	49.67	6.01	4.99	1.76		12.76	300.51	0.02	300.53	1,113.60	402.88	18.35	1,425.17	96
7. 1/2 C	30.71	1.97	32.68	3.83	5.99	2.11		11.93	191.97	0.02	191.99	727.39	280.41	12.02	956.95	90.20
8. P	28.80			3.60					180.00			678.00	216.00	10.80	830.60	100
9. C	67.19	4.17	71.36	8.40	12.49	4.47	30.43	55.79	420.00	0.59	420.59	1,521.65	609.79	26.15	2,359.04	82.10
10. P	19.49			2.40					120.00			432.00	144.00	7.02	554.60	100
11. C	36.55	1.97	38.52	4.55	5.99	2.11	8.11	20.76	227.83	0.02	227.85	860.10	324.65	14.20	1,195.20	88.10
12. C	36.77	1.97	38.74	4.59	5.99	2.11	5.99	18.68	279.87	0.02	279.89	863.85	325.90	14.34	1,386.40	80.25
13. C	54.30	2.05	56.35	6.78	7.60	2.21	20.28	36.87	339.43	0.03	339.46	1,230.45	418.22	20.45	1,861.28	84.10
14. C	61.44	1.97	63.41	7.68	5.99	2.11	12.17	27.95	384.00	0.02	384.02	1,418.70	510.85	23.09	1,955.60	90.81
15. C	68.08	6.82	74.90	8.51	20.28	7.30	20.28	56.37	425.50	0.97	426.47	1,607.18	683.35	26.12	2,487.01	83.04
16. C	63.36	1.97	65.33	6.33	10.14	2.11	20.28	38.86	396.04	0.02	396.06	1,052.79	389.12	17.86	2,163.69	86.92
17. C	84.75	3.94	88.69	10.59	10.14	4.22	15.21	40.76	529.71	0.04	529.75	1,979.25	735.54	32.68	2,816.25	90.60
18. C	61.43	2.50	63.93	7.67	7.60	2.68	15.21	33.16	383.96	0.04	384.00	1,438.39	527.66	23.71	1,998.75	93.70
19. P	69.11			8.63					431.95			1,555.03	518.34	25.91	1,995.54	100
20. P	9.05			1.13					56.61			203.79	67.93	3.36	261.50	100
21. P	18.10			2.26					113.22			407.58	135.86	6.72	523.00	100
22. P	60.36			7.54					377.78			1,358.20	452.73	22.63	1,742.98	100
23. C	67.32			8.41	4.99				420.80							

NOTE: The use of grams for energy-giving elements (proteins, lipids, glucides) and milligrams for the trace elements (phosphorus, calcium, iron) follow the tables indicating the composition of foods by Mme. L. Randoin. (Cf. her book *Vues actuelles sur le problème de l'alimentation avec tables de composition des aliments* [Paris, 1937]; Raymond Lalanne, *L'alimentation humaine*, new ed., Collection "Que sais-je?" [Paris, 1967].) The figures given apply to the edible part of foodstuffs, but in the past this term covered a great deal.

serious, for the work in the field required great expenditures of physical strength and the body was ill prepared to withstand the rigors of winter, since the houses were poorly heated, if at all. Was not the best way to fight the cold to take refuge in the stables and to share the warmth given off by the animals and thus to save on the precious wood?

3. Glucides, or sugars, are the source of muscular energy. The minimum of 40 g. was always exceeded by a wide margin, and glucides were the only source of energy furnished in sufficient quantity by this diet—but was this enough to compensate for its deficiencies?

The daily food intake must also furnish the organism certain trace elements or mineral salts, among them phosphorus and calcium. They are sometimes referred to as building blocks, since they are essential to the healthy development of the skeleton and the teeth, and they must be properly balanced: for the adult, the correct ratio between calcium and phosphorus (Ca/P) is between 0.6 and 0.8; for the pregnant woman, it is between 1 and 1.2; and for the child, who needs them for growth and the completion of the bone structure, it is between 1.2 and 1.5. Here again, in all the complete rations of Table 3, this ratio is between 0.32 and 0.43; hence an excess of phosphorus and a very pronounced deficiency of calcium, which was not compensated by an intake of vitamin D either, since milk products were consumed in very small quantities. All of this caused a great many bone diseases such as rickets, scoliosis, and frequent cases of bow legs, not to mention the early decay of the teeth, which were prematurely reduced to a few loose stumps blackened by chewing tobacco and ignorance of dental hygiene. As late as between the two world wars, many dentists of the Lozère[24] warned against this lack of calcium in the diet, some very limited progress since the eighteenth century not withstanding.

24. I am especially thinking of Dr. Charles Morel, Sr., president of the Société des Sciences, Lettres et Arts de la Lozère. Deceased not long ago (December, 1968), he was a great expert on the Lozère. He honored me with his friendship and had urged me to write the present article in the summer of 1968. I respectfully salute his memory here.

Insufficient amounts of calories, fats, and certain vitamins; deficiencies in animal proteins; a monotonous diet based almost exclusively on bread—all of this adds up to a rather unsatisfactory nutritional balance sheet. And even this represents only an average—arbitrary and misleading, since all averages for the rations stipulated in these pensions were not the same every year or even in the course of any given year. To use a well-known biblical image, we might say that there were "fat" and "lean cows"; the "lean cows," by far the most common, can be found first of all in the years of shortage that brought great hardship to the population. There was little grain, and only private charity organized by the church and sometimes assisted by the public authorities averted full-scale famine. After the disastrous harvest of 1693, for example, the estates of the Gévaudan voted a public loan of 30,000 livres "to be used for the purchase of grain in Lower Languedoc and for transportation to the towns of Mende and Langogne, where it will be distributed to the inhabitants of those parishes where the shortage is most severe" (March, 1694); at the same time, Msgr. Piencourt, the Bishop of Mende, asked the parish priests to report on the stocks of grain available in their parishes.[25] A great many of the responses to this episcopal inquiry were of the following nature: "No old grain." "There is not enough rye for seed." "The harvest has been so bad that we do not believe there is enough [grain] to sustain the parish for more than three or four months." "The inhabitants are so destitute that they are unable to buy any grain. . . ." The low tax rate confirms these statements. Such calamities seem to be much rarer in the eighteenth century. Does this mean that the situation had really improved, or is it a matter of documentation? In any case, the end of spring and the early summer until the first haying continued to be very difficult for man and beast: pantries, barns, and storage bins were almost empty, especially if the winter had been unusually long and hard. During this period before the new harvest (called

---

25. Cf. B. Bardy, "Statistiques économiques et agricoles en Gévaudan à la fin du XVIIe siècle," *Revue de Gévaudan, des Causses et des Cévennes*, 1958, pp. 71–90.

the *soudure*), people must have often left the table hungry and everyone was anxiously awaiting the new harvest "under the hand of the Good Lord" (reply of the parish of Canilhac to Msgr. de Piencourt, 1694). This is why the following statement is found in a considerable number of wills and marriage contracts: "There is enough grain to feed the household (or the family) until the next harvest," a statement that seems to imply that this was not necessarily the case. Also, many debts and mortgages on land and livestock were contracted in order to pay for the purchase of grain that the family needed to keep going. Most of the notarial documents relating to such debts and mortgages are dated in April, May, June, July. . . .

After the "lean cows," there were the "fat cows," but they were comparatively rare. These were occasions of feasting carried to the point of indigestion, as if the need for some kind of compensation and liberation—analogous to what might form the poor peasant's attitude toward money—led to excessive eating and drinking after prolonged periods of privation. Such brief interludes, such celebrations of the senses interrupting the oppressive monotony of everyday life, were, of course, also part of family celebrations such as baptisms and marriages.[26] Here the emotional nature of the occasion, the pleasure of seeing old friends, the desire to impress and outdo one's neighbors with the number of invited guests and the luxuries of the table, outweighed the usual acquisitiveness.

The end of the harvest was an occasion for great feasts. These brought together the master of the house and his family, the neighbors who had helped with the work, the mowers who were recruited in the region, and the teams (*colles*) of harvest

---

26. And even deaths: as in many other rural areas of France, the funeral banquet brought together all those who had come to the burial or to the novaine mass. These meals were surprisingly opulent, and the atmosphere in which they took place was quite relaxed, almost joyful. Should this be considered a vestige of paganism?

Travelers and passing guests were also treated very well: the best provisions from the storeroom were brought out for them, and one of the children was sent to sleep in the barn. . . . The peasant of the Gévaudan knew how to receive guests: antique hospitality was being perpetuated here.

hands who came up from Languedoc and were hired just before the harvest. After tenacious haggling with the "masters" over the wages to be paid, the hiring took place at something resembling a slave market in such towns as Châteauneuf-de-Randon. The spirited gaiety of these meals was reminiscent of the harvest meal described in Canto VII of Frederic Mistral's *Mireille*. Fresh roasted meat (quite an unusual luxury) was eaten, for on this occasion one or two sheep were killed and roasted on a spit outdoors; wine flowed generously and turned many a head that had not often tasted it; dancing the *bourrée* ended the festivities except for those who engaged in amorous pursuits in some discreet nook or cranny. . . .

And every year between December and March during the hardest time of winter, the "liturgy" of the *cochonailles* brightened the life of the peasant. This was the killing of the pig followed by the preparation of the meat (lard, ham, smoked and dry sausage) destined to feed the household in the months to come. The actual slaughtering of the pig was always done outdoors in front of the house no matter how hard the frost or how strong the gale. Amidst a cacophony of piercing squeals and grunts, the hapless pig, solidly held down by three or four strong neighbors, had its throat cut. It was then bled, and every last drop of it was saved. Afterward, the skin was cleaned by singeing it with wads of burning straw and scraping it with long, well-sharpened knives. After the carcass was cleaned in this fashion, it was brought indoors. Now the long and involved preparation could begin with the help of friends, relations, and experts in the art of meat processing. The smoked and dry sausages to be served to the mowers and field hands during the harvest were made first; they also appeared on the family table on very special occasions, as did the ham, which was salted, along with the lard,[27] somewhat later.

The blood and the fresh meat also had to be used. The blood was made into blood pudding and consumed on the spot. The

---

27. In Occitan, the language to which the dialect of the Lozère is closely related, the word for lard is *bacou*. Cf. the modern word *bacon*.

fresh meat was salted so that it could be kept for a month or two; it was then used for preparing *"maouchos."* This was done by digging out cabbages that had been buried before the onset of cold weather in "furrows," rudimentary kinds of silos where the cabbages had been blanched. These were boiled and mixed with the salted pork meat; then this stuffing was pressed into a piece of pork gut by means of an instrument ending in a long funnel called an *embuco* or *embuque*. This process yielded a cabbage sausage (*"maoucho"*) highly appreciated in those frugal days. The same was true of the *"tripoux,"* which are now being rediscovered by city people. These were pork intestines, finely chopped and tied together in small bundles, highly seasoned with salt and pepper, and simmered for an entire day.

These preparations, spaced out over several weeks, brought together many people, if only neighbors and relatives. They were the occasion for joyful revels. This was something to fill empty days and boost morales. It sustained village solidarity in the face of the rigors of winter as snow was beating against the tiny windows of the house, as the storm made the beams groan, as clouds spread their lugubrious shroud over the mountains, and as the terrible blizzard created huge snow drifts isolating the village and burying foolhardy or lost travelers. Here was a veritable "communion," for everyone felt less helpless before nature's winter furies. . . . It was not a matter of just eating good food, it was gluttony. If there had been any money for wine, it now flowed freely. Spirits rose, tongues were loosened, and in the long evenings a whole fund of stories, legends, and beliefs (some still steeped in pagan notions) from local folklore was transmitted not without elaboration and adaptation. Exceptionally rich food, accompanied by equally exceptional libations, to which the organism was not accustomed, imparted to some a surplus of vitality. Since this vitality could not be used for work in the fields, it was expended in conjugal intimacy in which couples enthusiastically engaged in the "sweet and delightful games of love." A sampling of data[28] now under way in the

---

28. Cf. a forthcoming article of mine.

parishes of Allenc and Chasseradès seems to indicate a very clear-cut rise in conceptions during the slaughtering period.

However, none of this is grounds for illusion. The "fat cows" represented only very short moments, and the peasant of the Gévaudan was far more familiar with the "lean cows"—in other words, with malnutrition on top of a chronically inadequate diet. What were the physiological consequences of this situation? For the answer to this question, we are unfortunately reduced to conjectures, hypotheses, and intuition, for over long periods of time the local authorities seem to have given very little thought to the state of the people's health. Before 1870, the minutes of the draft boards deal only in generalities; they do, however, call attention to the short stature and the bow legs of many of the recruits.[29]

Wills rather frequently mentioned crippled and deformed children unable to take care of their own needs. There is no proof, but would not these, in many cases, be individuals suffering from rickets and scrofula brought about by a deficient diet? And as for the abnormally high number of young mothers dying in childbirth or a few days or weeks after the birth of their child, was this strictly a matter of poor hygiene and poor prenatal care (under the best of circumstances a local matron was called in, and although she was called a midwife, her qualifications and competence are certainly open to doubt)? Or did chronic malnutrition make it impossible for the young mother (who worked, as usual, without sparing herself to the very end of her pregnancy) to resist the added stress of the delivery? These two causes, compounded in some cases by a somewhat delicate constitution, must often have come together. It should be noted that such deaths were especially frequent in the difficult period before the new harvest. This time of the year, as well as the depth of winter (January–March), was also the time when, in certain years, waves of mortality thinned out many a village and hamlet, and at such times no one was spared: men, women, old people, adults, children. Some of these "mortalities" can be

---

29. Service historique de l'état-major de l'armée, Vincennes, Ser. x5 (57–67).

explained by bad harvests in the previous year, resulting in short supplies of food resources: this was the case at Chasseradès and Belvezet (an annex of Chasseradès) in 1783–84. Others can be laid to the length and unusual rigor of the winter (Allenc, 1768–9; Saint-Jean-la-Foulhouze, 1780–81). But in all cases, malnutrition must have played a part, despite the feasts at slaughtering time. Another cause was the scarcity of heating fuel.

However, given the present state of documentation, all these questions can only be answered in a very approximate fashion.

One last problem deserves to be considered. Were the amounts stipulated in these food pensions determined, to a certain degree, by the economic position of the testators or of the parents of the future spouses? If this were the case, the smallest pensions, and especially the incomplete ones, would attest to the poverty of the contracting parties; conversely, the more substantial pensions would be granted by, and destined for, people in better circumstances. It is true that pension no. 17, the most copious, was destined for the wife of a testator who left a *légitime* of 1,500 livres to each of his two children, a son and a daughter. However, pension no. 9 appears in a marriage contract by which the future spouses together brought 350 livres worth of *cabaux*, a relatively modest sum, into the marriage. Pension no. 16 was granted by the will of a testator who left only a 400-livre *légitime* to each of his two daughters. On the other hand, the partial pension no. 2 is part of a marriage contract giving the bride a dowry of 889 livres 15 sols, quite a respectable sum. Pension no. 21, the most meager after no. 20, was granted by a testator who willed a *légitime* of 1,100 livres to an unborn posthumous child. Perhaps he thought that his widow would remarry soon, thus assuring her livelihood. . . . As for pension no. 3, it is part of a marriage contract that clearly states that the future husband will bring 800 livres into the marriage. . . .

In conclusion, while it is possible, indeed certain, that the financial position of the contracting parties determined the amounts of many of these food pensions, this is not true in every case, so that a direct correlation between these two factors can not be established.

One fundamental question arises at the end of this investigation: What interest does this research on diets of the past have for history in general? It shows once again, as previous research in similar areas has done, that if such a study is rooted in a thorough understanding of a region (and it must be an understanding from the "inside," not that of a hurried investigator who just stops by), it will open up new vistas not only in social and economic history, but also, and above all, in the history of "mentalities," behavior, and attitudes toward life in general. The history of diet can be one of the most valuable building blocks for social psychology. Understood in this fashion, it gives a new dimension to historical research.

In a more restricted sense, the history of diet gives eloquent testimony to the fundamental and permanent conservatism of the Gévaudan. Having preserved, until very recently, its personality in every aspect of life, its conservatism has made this *pagus* a veritable living museum, a conservatory of France's agrarian past.[30]

---

30. It is to be hoped that the necessary adaptation of the region to modern life (which is under way) will not deprive it of its substance and will not alter the unique, engaging, even exemplary traits it has preserved. These are very happily manifested in its inhabitants, whose sociability, quickness, and open-mindedness, already quite meridonal in character, temper the heaviness, stodginess, and acquisitiveness of nearby Auvergne.

Toward a Psychosociology of Contemporary Food Consumption

ROLAND BARTHES

The inhabitants of the United States consume almost twice as much sugar as the French.[1] Such a fact is usually a concern of economics and politics. But this is by no means all. One needs only to take the step from sugar as merchandise, an abstract item in accounts, to sugar as food, a concrete item that is "eaten" rather than "consumed," to get an inkling of the (probably unexplored) depth of the phenomenon. For the Americans must do something with all that sugar. And as a matter of fact, anyone who has spent time in the United States knows that sugar permeates a considerable part of American cooking; that it saturates ordinarily sweet foods, such as pastries; makes for a great variety of sweets served, such as ice creams, jellies, syrups; and is used in many dishes that French people do not sweeten, such as meats, fish, salads, and relishes. This is something that would be of interest to scholars in fields other than economics, to the psychosociologist, for example, who will have

SOURCE: "Vers une psycho-sociologie de l'alimentation moderne" by Roland Barthes, in *Annales: Économies, Sociétés, Civilisations* no. 5 (September–October, 1961), pp. 977–986. Reprinted by permission of *Annales*.

1. Annual sugar consumption in the United States is 43 kg. per person; in France, 25 kg. per person.

something to say about the presumably invariable relation between standard of living and sugar consumption. (But is this relation really invariable today? And if so, why?)[2] It could be of interest to the historian also, who might find it worthwhile to study the ways in which the use of sugar evolved as part of American culture (the influence of Dutch and German immigrants who were used to "sweet-salty" cooking?). Nor is this all. Sugar is not just a foodstuff, even when it is used in conjunction with other foods; it is, if you will, an "attitude," bound to certain usages, certain "protocols," that have to do with more than food. Serving a sweet relish or drinking a Coca-Cola with a meal are things that are confined to eating habits proper; but to go regularly to a dairy bar, where the absence of alcohol coincides with a great abundance of sweet beverages, means more than to consume sugar; through the sugar, it also means to experience the day, periods of rest, traveling, and leisure in a specific fashion that is certain to have its impact on the American. For who would claim that in France wine is only wine? Sugar or wine, these two superabundant substances are also institutions. And these institutions necessarily imply a set of images, dreams, tastes, choices, and values. I remember an American hit song: *Sugar Time*. Sugar is a time, a category of the world.[3]

I have started out with the example of the American use of sugar because it permits us to get outside of what we, as Frenchmen, consider "obvious." For we do not see our own food or, worse, we assume that it is insignificant. Even—or perhaps especially—to the scholar, the subject of food connotes triviality or guilt.[4] This may explain in part why the psychosociology of French eating habits is still approached only indirectly and in passing when more weighty subjects, such as life-styles, budgets, and advertising, are under discussion. But at least the

2. F. Charny, *Le sucre*, Collection "Que sais-je?" (Paris: P. U. F., 1950), p. 8.
3. I do not wish to deal here with the problem of sugar "metaphors" or paradoxes, such as the "sweet" rock singers or the sweet milk beverages of certain "toughs."
4. Motivation studies have shown that food advertising openly based on enjoyment are apt to fail, since they make the reader feel guilty (J. Marcus-Steiff, *Les études de motivation* [Paris: Hermann, 1961], pp. 44–45).

sociologists, the historians of the present—since we are talking only about contemporary eating habits here—and the economists are already aware that there is such a thing.

Thus P. H. Chombart de Lauwe has made an excellent study of the behavior of French working-class families with respect to food. He was able to define areas of frustration and to outline some of the mechanisms by which needs are transformed into values, necessities into alibis.[5] In her book *Le mode de vie des familles bourgeoises de 1873 à 1953*, M. Perrot came to the conclusion that economic factors played a less important role in the changes that have taken place in middle-class food habits in the last hundred years than changing tastes; and this really means ideas, especially about nutrition.[6] Finally, the development of advertising has enabled the economists to become quite conscious of the ideal nature of consumer goods; by now everyone knows that the product as bought—that is, experienced—by the consumer is by no means the real product; between the former and the latter there is a considerable production of false perceptions and values. By being faithful to a certain brand and by justifying this loyalty with a set of "natural" reasons, the consumer gives diversity to products that are technically so identical that frequently even the manufacturer cannot find any differences. This is notably the case with most cooking oils.[7]

It is obvious that such deformations or reconstructions are not only the manifestation of individual, anomic prejudices, but also elements of a veritable collective imagination showing the outlines of a certain mental framework. All of this, we might say, points to the (necessary) widening of the very notion of food. For what is food? It is not only a collection of products that can

---

5. P. H. Chombart de Lauve, *La vie quotidienne des familles ouvrières* (Paris: C.N.R.S., 1956).

6. Marguerite Perrot, *Le mode de vie des familles bourgeoises, 1873–1953* (Paris: Colin, 1961). "Since the end of the nineteenth century, there has been a very marked evolution in the dietary habits of the middle-class families we have investigated in this study. This evolution seems related, not to a change in the standard of living, but rather to a transformation of individual tastes under the influence of a greater awareness of the rules of nutrition" (p. 292).

7. J. Marcus-Steiff, *Les études de motivation*, p. 28.

be used for statistical or nutritional studies. It is also, and at the same time, a system of communication, a body of images, a protocol of usages, situations, and behavior. Information about food must be gathered wherever it can be found: by direct observation in the economy, in techniques, usages, and advertising; and by indirect observation in the mental life of a given society.[8] And once these data are assembled, they should no doubt be subjected to an internal analysis that should try to establish what is significant about the way in which they have been assembled before any economic or even ideological determinism is brought into play. I should like to give a brief outline of what such an analysis might be.

When he buys an item of food, consumes it, or serves it, modern man does not manipulate a simple object in a purely transitive fashion; this item of food sums up and transmits a situation; it constitutes an information; it signifies. That is to say that it is not just an indicator of a set of more or less conscious motivations, but that it is a real sign, perhaps the functional unit of a system of communication. By this I mean not only the elements of *display* in food, such as foods involved in rites of hospitality,[9] for all food serves as a sign among the members of a given society. As soon as a need is satisfied by standardized production and consumption, in short, as soon as it takes on the characteristics of an institution, its function can no longer be dissociated from the sign of that function. This is true for clothing;[10] it is also true for food. No doubt, food is, anthropologically speaking (though very much in the abstract), the first need; but ever since man has ceased living off wild berries, this need has been highly structured. Substances, techniques of preparation, habits, all become part of a system of differences in

---

8. On the latest techniques of investigation, see again J. Marcus-Steiff, *Les études de motivation*.

9. Yet on this point alone, there are many known facts that should be assembled and systematized: cocktail parties, formal dinners, degrees and kinds of display by way of food according to the different social groups.

10. R. Barthes, "Le bleu est à la mode cette année: Note sur la recherche des unités signifiantes dans le vêtement de mode," *Revue française de sociologie* 1 (1960): 147–162.

signification; and as soon as this happens, we have communication by way of food. For the fact that there is communication is proven, not by the more or less vague consciousness that its users may have of it, but by the ease with which all the facts concerning food form a structure analogous to other systems of communication.[11] People may very well continue to believe that food is an immediate reality (necessity or pleasure), but this does not prevent it from carrying a system of communication: it would not be the first thing that people continue to experience as a simple function at the very moment when they constitute it into a sign.

If food is a system, what might be its constituent units? In order to find out, it would obviously be necessary to start out with a complete inventory of all we know of the food in a given society (products, techniques, habits), and then to subject these facts to what the linguists call transformational analysis, that is, to observe whether the passage from one fact to another produces a difference in signification. Here is an example: the changeover from ordinary bread to *pain de mie* involves a difference in what is signified: the former signifies day-to-day life, the latter a party. Similarly, in contemporary terms, the changeover from white to brown bread corresponds to a change in what is signified in social terms, because, paradoxically, brown bread has become a sign of refinement. We are therefore justified in considering the varieties of bread as units of signification—at least these varieties—for the same test can also show that there are insignificant varieties as well, whose use has nothing to do with a collective institution, but simply with individual taste. In this manner, one could, proceeding step by step, make a compendium of the differences in signification regulating the system of our food. In other words, it would be a matter of separating the significant from the insignificant and then of reconstructing the differential system of signification by constructing, if I may

---

11. I am using the word *structure* in the sense that it has in linguistics: "an autonomous entity of internal dependencies" (L. Hjelnislev, *Essais linguistiques* [Copenhagen, 1959], p. 1).

be permitted to use such a metaphor, a veritable grammar of foods.

It must be added that the units of our system would probably coincide only rarely with the products in current use in the economy. Within French society, for example, bread as such does not constitute a signifying unit: in order to find these we must go further and look for certain of its varieties. In other words, these signifying units are more subtle than the commercial units and, above all, they have to do with subdivisions with which production is not concerned, so that the sense of the subdivision can differentiate a single product. Thus it is not at the level of its preparation and use that the sense of a food item is elaborated, but at the level of its preparation and use. There is perhaps no brute item of food that signifies anything in itself, except for a few deluxe items such as salmon, caviar, truffles, and so on, whose preparation is less important than their absolute cost.

If the units of our system of food are not the *products* of our economy, can we at least have some preliminary idea of what they might be? In the absence of a systematic inventory, we may risk a few hypotheses. A study by P. F. Lazarsfeld[12] (it is old, concerned with particulars, and I cite it only as an example) has shown that certain sensorial "tastes" can vary according to the income level of the social groups interviewed: lower-income persons like sweet chocolates, smooth materials, strong perfumes; the upper classes, on the other hand, prefer bitter substances, irregular materials, and light perfumes. To remain within the area of food, we can see that signification (which, itself, refers to a twofold social phenomenon: upper classes/lower classes) does not involve kinds of products, but flavors: *sweet* and *bitter* make up the opposition in signification, so that we must place certain units of the system of food on that level. We can imagine other classes of units, for example, opposite substances such as dry, creamy, watery ones, which im-

---

12. P. F. Lazarsfeld, "The Psychological Aspect of Market Research," *Harvard Business Review* 13 (1934): 54–71.

mediately show their great psychoanalytical potential (and it is obvious that if the subject of food had not been so trivialized and invested with guilt, it could easily be subjected to the kind of "poetic" analysis that G. Bachelard applied to language). As for what is considered tasty, C. Lévi-Strauss has already shown that this might very well constitute a class of oppositions that refers to national characters (French versus English cuisine, French versus Chinese or German cuisine, and so on).[13]

Finally, one can imagine opposites that are even more encompassing, but also more subtle. Why not speak, if the facts are sufficiently numerous and sufficiently clear, of a certain "spirit" of food, if I may be permitted to use this romantic term? By this I mean that a coherent set of food traits and habits can constitute a complex but homogeneous dominant feature useful for defining a general system of tastes and habits. This "spirit" brings together different units (such as flavor or substance), forming a composite unit with a single signification, somewhat analogous to the suprasegmental prosodic units of language. I should like to suggest here two very different examples. The ancient Greeks unified in a single (euphoric) notion the ideas of succulence, brightness, and moistness, and they called it γάνος. Honey had γάνος, and wine was the γάνος of the vineyard.[14] Now this would certainly be a signifying unit if we were to establish the system of food of the Greeks, even though it does not refer to any particular item. And here is another example, modern this time. In the United States, the Americans seem to oppose the category of sweet (and we have already seen to how many different varieties of foods this applies) with an equally general category that is not, however, that of salty—understandably so, since their food is salty and sweet to begin with —but that of *crisp* or *crispy*. *Crisp* designates everything that crunches, crackles, grates, sparkles, from potato chips to certain brands of beer; *crisp*—and this shows that the unit of food can overthrow logical categories—*crisp* may be applied to a product

---

13. C. Lévi-Strauss, *Anthropologie structurale* (Paris: Plon, 1958), p. 99.
14. H. Jeanmaire, *Dionysos* (Paris: Payot), p. 510.

just because it is ice cold, to another because it is sour, to a third because it is brittle. Quite obviously, such a notion goes beyond the purely physical nature of the product: *crispness* in a food designates an almost magical quality, a certain briskness and sharpness, as opposed to the soft, soothing character of sweet foods.

Now then, how will we use the units established in this manner? We will use them to reconstruct systems, syntaxes ("menus"), and styles ("diets")[15] no longer in an empirical but in a semantic way—in a way, that is, that will enable us to compare them to each other. We now must show, not that which is, but that which signifies. Why? Because we are interested in human communication and because communication always implies a system of signification, that is, a body of discrete signs standing out from a mass of indifferent materials. For this reason, sociology must, as soon as it deals with cultural "objects" such as clothing, food, and—not quite as clearly—housing, structure these objects before trying to find out what society does with them. For what society does with them is precisely to structure them in order to make use of them.

To what, then, can these significations of food refer? As I have already pointed out, they refer not only to display,[16] but to a much larger set of themes and situations. One could say that an entire "world" (social environment) is present in and signified by food. Today we have a tool with which to isolate these themes and situations, namely, advertising. There is no question that advertising provides only a projected image of reality; but the sociology of mass communication has become increasingly inclined to think that large-scale advertising, even though technically the work of a particular group, reflects the collective

---

15. In a semantic analysis, vegetarianism, for example (at least at the level of specialized restaurants), would appear as an attempt to copy the appearance of meat dishes by means of a series of artifices that are somewhat similar to "costume jewelry" in clothing, at least the jewelry that is meant to be seen as such.

16. The idea of social *display* must not be associated purely and simply with vanity; the analysis of motivation, when conducted by indirect questioning, reveals that worry about appearances is part of an extremely subtle reaction and that social strictures are very strong, even with respect to food.

psychology much more than it shapes it. Furthermore, studies of motivation are now so advanced that it is possible to analyze cases in which the response of the public is negative. (I already mentioned the feelings of guilt fostered by an advertising for sugar which emphasized pure enjoyment. It was bad advertising, but the response of the public was nonetheless psychologically most interesting.)

A rapid glance at food advertising permits us rather easily, I think, to identify three groups of themes. The first of these assigns to food a function that is, in some sense, commemorative: food permits a person (and I am here speaking of French themes) to partake each day of the national past. In this case, this historical quality is obviously linked to food techniques (preparation and cooking). These have long roots, reaching back to the depth of the French past. They are, we are told, the repository of a whole experience, of the accumulated wisdom of our ancestors. French food is never supposed to be innovative, except when it rediscovers long-forgotten secrets. The historical theme, which was so often sounded in our advertising, mobilizes two different values: on the one hand, it implies an aristocratic tradition (dynasties of manufacturers, *moutarde du Roy*, the Brandy of Napoleon); on the other hand, food frequently carries notions of representing the flavorful survival of an old, rural society that is itself highly idealized.[17] In this manner, food brings the memory of the soil into our very contemporary life; hence the paradoxical association of gastronomy and industrialization in the form of canned "gourmet dishes." No doubt the myth of French cooking abroad (or as expressed to foreigners) strengthens this "nostalgic" value of food considerably; but since the French themselves actively participate in this myth (especially when traveling), it is fair to say that through his food the Frenchman experiences a certain national continuity. By way of a thousand detours, food permits him to insert himself

---

17. The expression *cuisine bourgeoise*, used at first in a literal, then in a metaphoric way, seems to be gradually disappearing; while the "peasant stew" is periodically featured in the photographic pages of the major ladies' magazines.

daily into his own past and to believe in a certain culinary "being" of France.[18]

A second group of values concerns what we might call the anthropological situation of the French consumer. Motivation studies have shown that feelings of inferiority were attached to certain foods and that people therefore abstained from them.[19] For example, there are supposed to be masculine and feminine kinds of food. Furthermore, visual advertising makes it possible to associate certain kinds of foods with images connoting a sublimated sexuality. In a certain sense, advertising eroticizes food and thereby transforms our consciousness of it, bringing it into a new sphere of situations by means of a pseudocausal relationship.

Finally, a third area of consciousness is constituted by a whole set of ambiguous values of a somatic as well as psychic nature, clustering around the concept of *health*. In a mythical way, health is indeed a simple relay midway between the body and the mind; it is the alibi food gives to itself in order to signify materially a pattern of immaterial realities. Health is thus experienced through food only in the form of "conditioning," which implies that the body is able to cope with a certain number of day-to-day situations. Conditioning originates with the body but goes beyond it. It produces *energy* (sugar, the "powerhouse of foods," at least in France, maintains an "uninterrupted flow of energy"; margarine "builds solid muscles"; coffee "dissolves fatigue"); *alertness* ("Be alert with Lustucru") and *relaxation* (coffee, mineral water, fruit juices, Coca-Cola, and so on). In this manner, food does indeed retain its physiological function by giving strength to the organism, but this strength is immediately sublimated and placed into a specific situation (I shall come back to this in a moment). This situation may be one

---

18. The exotic nature of food can, of course, be a value, but in the French public at large, it seems limited to coffee (tropical) and pasta (Italian).

19. This would be the place to ask just what is meant by "strong" food. Obviously, there is no psychic quality inherent in the thing itself. A food becomes "masculine" as soon as women, children, and old people, for nutritional (and thus fairly historical) reasons, do not consume it.

of conquest (alertness, aggressiveness) or a response to the stress of modern life (relaxation). No doubt, the existence of such themes is related to the spectacular development of the science of nutrition, to which, as we have seen, one historian unequivocally attributes the evolution of food budgets over the last fifty years. It seems, then, that the acceptance of this new value by the masses has brought about a new phenomenon, which must be the first item of study in any psychosociology of food: it is what might be called nutritional consciousness. In the developed countries, food is henceforth *thought out*, not by specialists, but by the entire public, even if this thinking is done within a framework of highly mythical notions. Nor is this all. This nutritional rationalizing is aimed in a specific direction. Modern nutritional science (at least according to what can be observed in France) is not bound to any moral values, such as asceticism, wisdom, or purity,[20] but on the contrary, to values of *power*. The energy furnished by a consciously worked out diet is mythically directed, it seems, toward an adaptation of man to the modern world. In the final analysis, therefore, a representation of contemporary existence is implied in the consciousness we have of the function of our food.[21]

For, as we said before, food serves as a sign not only for themes, but also for situations; and this, all told, means for a way of life that is emphasized, much more than expressed, by it. To eat is a behavior that develops beyond its own ends, replacing, summing up, and signaling other behaviors, and it is precisely for these reasons that it is a sign. What are these other behaviors? Today, we might say all of them: activity, work, sports, effort, leisure, celebration—every one of these situations is expressed through food. We might almost say that this "polysemia" of food characterizes modernity; in the past, only festive occasions were signalized by food in any positive and organized manner. But today, work also has its own kind of

---

20. We need only to compare the development of vegetarianism in England and France.

21. Right now, in France, there is a conflict between traditional (gastronomic) and modern (nutritional) values.

food (on the level of a sign, that is): energy-giving and light food is experienced as the very sign of, rather than only a help toward, participation in modern life. The snack bar not only responds to a new need, it also gives a certain dramatic expression to this need and shows those who frequent it to be modern men, managers who exercise power and control over the extreme rapidity of modern life. Let us say that there is an element of "Napoleonism" in this ritually condensed, light, and rapid kind of eating. On the level of institutions, there is also the business lunch, a very different kind of thing, which has become commercialized in the form of special menus: here, on the contrary, the emphasis is placed on comfort and long discussions; there even remains a trace of the mythical conciliatory power of conviviality. Hence, the business lunch emphasizes the gastronomic, and under certain circumstances traditional, value of the dishes served and uses this value to stimulate the euphoria needed to facilitate the transaction of business. Snack bar and business lunch are two very closely related work situations, yet the food connected with them signalizes their differences in a perfectly readable manner. We can imagine many others that should be catalogued.

This much can be said already: today, at least in France, we are witnessing an extraordinary expansion of the areas associated with food: food is becoming incorporated into an ever-lengthening list of situations. This adaptation is usually made in the name of hygiene and better living, but in reality, to stress this fact once more, food is also charged with signifying the situation in which it is used. It has a twofold value, being nutrition as well as protocol, and its value as protocol becomes increasingly more important as soon as the basic needs are satisfied, as they are in France. In other words, we might say that in contemporary French society *food has a constant tendency to transform itself into situation*.

There is no better illustration for this trend than the advertising mythology about coffee. For centuries, coffee was considered a stimulant to the nervous system (recall that Michelet claimed that it led to the Revolution), but contemporary advertising, while not expressly denying this traditional function, paradoxically associates it more and more with images of "breaks," rest, and even relaxation. What is the reason for this shift? It is that coffee is felt to be not so much a substance[22] as a circumstance. It is the recognized occasion for interrupting work and using this respite in a precise protocol of taking sustenance. It stands to reason that if this transferral of the food substance to its use becomes really all-encompassing, the power of signification of food will be vastly increased. Food, in short, will lose in substance and gain in function; this function will be general and point to activity (such as the business lunch) or to times of rest (such as coffee); but since there is a very marked opposition between work and relaxation, the traditionally festive function of food is apt to disappear gradually, and society will arrange the signifying system of its food around two major focal points: on the one hand, activity (and no longer work), and on the other hand, leisure (no longer celebration). All of this goes to show, if indeed it needs to be shown, to what extent food is an organic system, organically integrated into its specific type of civilization.

---

22. It seems that this stimulating, re-energizing power is now assigned to sugar, at least in France.

The General Relationship between Diet and Industrialization

H. J. TEUTEBERG

Survey of Changes in the Margin of Food Supply and the Composition of Diet

The scattered literature on the history of nutrition in Germany in the eighteenth and nineteenth centuries provides certain factual data as well as some preliminary assumptions. Reliable quantification and generalization about nutrition in the various social classes for periods before the development of scientific statistics and empirical work in economics and sociology does not appear feasible. We neither know the quantity and quality of food consumption at all times and places in sufficient detail, nor are there any representative samples in a modern sense. Furthermore, these earlier centuries do not yield any usable criteria of social stratification for statistical and empirical analysis. The existing source material is insufficient for establishing exact differentiations among the dietary habits of the various strata of society. Thus a quantitatively reliable history of the standards of nutrition is possible only from the beginning of the twentieth

SOURCE: Chapter 3, part 1, of *Der Wandel der Nahrungsgewohnheiten unter dem Einfluss der Industrialisierung* by H. J. Teuteberg and G. Wiegelmann. Reprinted by permission of Vandenhoek & Ruprecht.

century. This situation is true for the entire history of consumption, of which the history of nutrition must be considered a part. If statistics on consumption occupied, until the end of the nineteenth century, a very modest place in comparison with those on production and trade, this fact does not indicate the lesser importance of consumption, but rather the specific difficulties of scientific data-gathering. For a long time it was considered impossible to attempt an exact numerical accounting of all the goods consumed in a given country and especially of the foods eaten. Bold estimates served only to make the few attempts at generalization unreliable and even to discredit the entire field of consumption statistics, including some valuable data contained in them.[1] This fact was no doubt one of the main obstacles to a more intensive study of the changes in the standard of nutrition and helps to explain why research in this field has, so far, been inadequate.

Today, however, we are likely to overlook the fact that the eighteenth and nineteenth centuries already had a wide variety of scattered local data, estimates based on per capita consumption, and other attempts at quantification that nutritional research in historical ethnology can henceforth no longer ignore. Inadequate, fragmentary, and varied though these recorded data may be, once they are sufficiently numerous, systematized, and converted into modern measures and nutritional units, it will at least be possible to establish relatively sure approximations of the great structural changes in the nutrition of a nation.

The historical calculations and estimations for the other branches of the economy, such as those made by Walter G. Hoffmann, Knut Borchart, and others, involved very similar methodological difficulties. There is no reason why the history of nutrition should not make similar preliminary attempts at quantification. These will certainly call for all kinds of manipula-

---

1. On this point, see the still interesting dissertation by the student of Conrad K. Apelt, *Konsumption der wichtigsten Kulturländer in den letzten Jahrzehnten* (Halle, 1899), pp. 1 ff. In this dissertation, all the important works of the older literature on consumption (McCulloch, Levi, Dieterici, Viebahn, Bienengräber, Block, Lexis, Mullhall, Scherzer, Neumann-Spallart) are listed and critically evaluated.

tion and "tricks" if source materials from the past are to be interpreted to arrive at an overall understanding. The research findings to date in historical standards of living in Great Britain have already shown that the cautious use of quantitative data yields far more exact results than deductive theories in these matters.[2] It is more than probable that especially in the field of nutritional history a number of scientific assumptions will have to be revised. There are strong indications that large areas of nutritional history are riddled with historical legends that are in great need of scientific historical treatment. As far as we can see, no monographic summary and interpretation of the older German consumption statistics has been attempted, with the exception of some studies of meat consumption by Gustav Schmoller and his disciples, so that there is an urgent need for research here. But in any case, empirically arrived at approximations based on primitive statistics are always preferable to speculative theories.[3] The early per capita statistics, based as they were on estimates and generalization from scattered data, yielded—to stress this once again—only a very rough and approximate pic-

2. For the more advanced historical research in Great Britain, see, among others: R. M. Hartwell, "The Rising Standard of Living in England, 1800–1850," *Economic History Review*, 2nd ser. 13 (1960–61): 397; T. S. Ashton, "The Standard of Living of the Workers in England, 1790–1830," *Journal of Economic History*, Suppl., 9 (1949): 19; E. J. Hobsbawm, "The British Standard of Living, 1790–1840," *Economic History Review*, 2nd ser. 10 (1957): 46; A. J. Taylor, "Progress and Poverty in Britain, 1780–1850," *History* 45 (1960): 16. . . . All of these articles have been translated [into German] and can be found in the volume edited by Wolfram Fischer and Georg Bajor, *Die Soziale Frage: Neuere Studien zur Lage der Fabrikarbeiter in den Frühphasen der Industrialisierung* (Stuttgart, 1967), pp. 51–158. The state of this historical debate is concisely summarized in Phyllis Deane, *The First Industrial Revolution* (Cambridge, 1965), pp. 237 ff.

3. The author arrived at these conclusions after a number of conversations with the German-American political economist Carl Landauer (Berkeley) and after becoming acquainted with the "school of new economic history." When the present study was being written, the collection of essays edited by Wolfram Fischer, *Wirtschaftliche und soziale Probleme der frühen Industrialisierung* (Berlin, 1968), had not yet been published. Very much in accordance with my own views, Fischer, in his introduction, urges German economic historians to make greater efforts than in the past to avail themselves of the original source materials for quantification, admittedly a particularly difficult task in the German case. I would certainly second Fischer's exhortation: "Let us not be afraid of theoretical political economy and statistics."

ture of actual food consumption. Rich and poor, children and old people, North and South, men and women, Jews and Catholics, were lumped together under an average figure. Nonetheless, these per capita figures must be considered indispensable tools for studying centuries that simply did not have any reliable general statistics. Accounts by knowledgeable contemporaries and closer observation of specific groups can be used to supplement and check the rough averages. The historian of nutrition will, of course, be interested in differentiating these rough approximations as much as possible, if his sources permit. But he will have to resign himself to working mostly with per capita figures for the periods prior to the end of the nineteenth century, when social consumption statistics become available.

Purposely disregarding short-term variations and regional differentiations, a long-range and general analysis of changes in the nutritional standards of Germany can be summarized as follows:

It appears that in all of Europe the margin of food supply became too narrow by the sixteenth century at the latest. The relatively high meat content of the diet, for example, which still existed in the late Middle Ages, was increasingly replaced by vegetable products in the subsequent centuries. This was a gradual process of "depecoration"—that is, increasing "meatlessness"—as it was called by the political economist Wilhelm Roscher, the first scholar to call attention to this phenomenon.[4] The consumption of butter, eggs, fowl, and wine—the latter displaced by the cheaper beer—also seems to have decreased since the late Middle Ages. A voluminous diet

---

4. Wilhelm Roscher, *Die Nationalökonomik des Ackerbaues und der verwandten Urproduktionen*, ed. Dade 13th ed., (Stuttgart and Berlin, 1913). Cf. also Gustav Schmoller, "Die historische Entwicklung des Fleischkonsums sowie der Vieh- und Fleischpreise in Deutschland," *Zeitschrift für die gesamte Staatswissenschaft* 27 (1871): 284–362; Wilhelm Abel, *Agrarkrisen und Agrarkonjunktur: Eine Geschichte der Land und Ernährungswirtschaft Mitteleuropas seit dem hohen Mittelalter*, 2nd ed. (Hamburg and Berlin, 1966), p. 236, particularly stresses the drop in real wages since the late Middle Ages.

that was low in fats and high in carbohydrates and "cheaper," despite the increasing general cost of foodstuffs, gradually displaced the previous diet, which had been more concentrated, richer in animal proteins, and more "expensive" per nutritional unit. But even though Germany in the nineteenth century experienced an unprecedented "population explosion" due to falling mortality rates, earlier and more numerous marriages, and a rise in real per capita incomes, the margin of food supply stopped shrinking. On the contrary, the per capita quantity of meat consumed rose about threefold between 1816 and 1914, thus reaching about one-half of the medieval meat consumption, which modern estimates place at about 100 kg. per year per person.[5] This plainly amounts to a reversal of the Malthusian theory, which, as we know, prophesied in 1798 that the population would rise in geometric progression (1, 4, 8, 16, and so on) while the productivity of the soil would rise in only arithmetic progression (1, 2, 3, 4, and so on), a prospect that was linked to a number of gloomy prospects for the economy and society. Robert Thomas Malthus, the English clergyman who had come to grips with this problem while studying the parish registers —at that time the only reliable population statistics, saw the land as a specifically limited commodity, by its very nature incapable of increase. By contrast, he saw man the consumer as capable of practically unlimited increase. The Malthusian theory (originally meant as a critique of the populationist theories of mercantilism) has always been reversible from a purely logical point of view: it is, after all, possible to view trained and rational human labor as a specifically limited commodity and nature's potential for producing food as virtually inexhaustible. In the face of the misery in present-day developing countries, the Malthusian theory that the production of food cannot keep up with uncontrolled human procreation is still widely accepted. What its proponents always fail to take into account is the fact that, on the one hand, the disproportional rise in population

---

5. Rudolf Martin, "Der Fleischverbrauch im Mittelalter und in der Gegenwart," *Preussische Jahrbücher* 82 (1895), pp. 308–342; Kurt Hintze, *Die Lage der ländlichen Arbeiter in Mecklenburg* (1894), p. 101; Abel, *Agrarkrisen*, p. 247.

will not continue once the process of industrialization is completed and, on the other, that the possibilities for food production have not yet been exhausted by any means. The production of artificial meat from synthetics, plantations of sea algae, artificial irrigation by means of solar or atomic energy, "chicken factories," new foods such as those developed for the use of astronauts, and frozen foods, are some examples. Histories of all industrial countries show that there are always two complementary tendencies: one that brings a rapid improvement in agricultural productivity, and one leading to a slower, arrested, or even reversed population growth, so that the Malthusian law is suspended. The history of nutrition in nineteenth-century Germany, insofar as it is known to us, confirms this reciprocal trend.

This is a rather important point to make, since we know that the Malthusian theory was a vital prerequisite for the formulation of the "law of diminishing returns" and the thesis of the "iron law of wages." After all, Karl Marx's predictions concerning the formation of an "industrial reserve army" and chronic underconsumption due to an increasing frequency of crisis within the capitalist economy are really nothing but variations of the old Malthusian skepticism about man's superiority over nature. Malthus saw man only as a passive consumer and failed to see his potential role as a creative producer, a potential that, to be sure, was still dormant in Malthus's day. But in the course of the nineteenth century, man's creative activity in the field of food production showed how relative the Malthusian categories are. In stark contrast to his pessimistic prognosis, food production could be increased more easily precisely because of the increase in the number of people.

If we disregard all temporary food crises and the extremely variable dietary habits of various social groups, regions, and so on, that frequently serve to obscure the larger secular trends, the findings of modern scholarship so far are perfectly clear. The nineteenth century as a whole shows an extremely rapid and effective improvement in the standard of nutrition that definitely did away with the age-old "soup-and-porridge standard."[6] Improvements in the consumption of individual foodstuffs that became visible in the long run coincided rather consistently with the beginning of industrialization—a fact that will have to be illustrated in greater detail—so that they must be understood as hitherto almost unexplored side effects of that great revolution. From this perspective, it appears that those historians who claim that the industrialization of the nineteenth century brought about a higher standard of living in general were correct.

So far, we still know relatively little about the changes in the use of individual food items, but we do know that man has always preferred a mixed diet. Neither a purely vegetable nor a purely meat diet has ever been adopted for very long. A purely vegetable diet has always been a necessity for the poor in times of scarcity. But it is a remarkable fact that the upper classes, who were not restricted in their choice of food, never lived on meat alone. People have always tried to eat a diet that is as digestible as possible, yet tasty, easy to obtain, and easy to prepare. By these criteria, meat proved to be superior to all other foodstuffs, since it is rich in protein, tasty, and easy to prepare in many different ways. The higher the level of civilization, the more varied the diet becomes. The nature of the soil, climate, tradition, religious beliefs; the general state of cultural development, understanding of physiological phenomena, level of education; and the state of the economy and technology must be considered the most important factors influencing this basic desire, but in various degrees at different times.

As at all times and in all countries, vegetable foods formed the mainstay of the diet in nineteenth-century Germany. Vegetables high in carbohydrates were supplemented to a greater or lesser extent by animal products of varying quantity and quality. A long-term overview suggests a gradual changeover from the above-mentioned voluminous and less palatable staples with high roughage content such as potatoes, bread, legumes and

---

6. Rudolf Braun, *Industrialisierung und Volksleben* (Zurich, 1960); Martin, "Fleischverbrauch."

vegetable fats, to more digestible, nutritious, and tastier products such as meat, sugar, white bread, and so forth. Thus there seems to be a trend away from vegetable to animal protein and a decrease of carbohydrates in favor of fats, which is a reversal of the movement in previous centuries since the end of the Middle Ages.[7] Here is an example to illustrate this trend briefly. In 1800, according to the calculations of the statistician Leopold Krug, 53 percent of the monetary value of the entire food sector of the Prussian economy was spent on grain, 23 percent on other vegetable products, and only 24 percent of all foodstuffs were of animal origin. Today, almost the reverse is true: 72 percent of agricultural production is concerned with animal products.[8]

Ever since the nineteenth century, there was a general desire to develop a more healthful, digestible and varied diet. There was a turn from rough, poorly prepared food and drink to a more refined and appealing diet. In the last one hundred years or so, all industrialized countries show basically the same changes. The consumption of fruit (including tropical and dried fruit), vegetables, meat, eggs, fats, and sugar is increasing, while that of potatoes, legumes, and grain is, in general, decreasing.[9] The consumption of fats has increased by about 50 percent, that of eggs by about 92 percent. The greatest increase occurred in the consumption of fruit, which rose by 156 percent. By contrast, the consumption of potatoes dropped by about 29 percent over the last fifty years, and that of grain by 30 percent. Butter as well has clearly lost importance in Germany, but this is not true in all industrial countries.[10] By contrast, the present-day developing countries clearly exhibit the nutritional

---

7. Alfred Lichtenfeld, *Die Geschichte der Ernährung* (Berlin, 1913); Adam Maurizio, *Die Geschichte unserer Pflanzennahrung von den Urzeiten bis zur Gegenwart* (Berlin, 1922).

8. Wilhelm Abel, *Geschichte der deutschen Landwirtschaft vom frühen Mittelalter bis zum 19. Jahrhundert* (Stuttgart, 1962), p. 300.

9. Hans Glatzel, *Altbekanntes und Neuerforschtes vom Essen*, 2nd ed. (Berlin, n.d.); Abel, *Agrarkrisen*, p. 247.

10. The rate of consumption of fruit and also of vegetables might be somewhat misleading, since we know practically nothing about per capita consumption in earlier times. Home garden production played a particularly important role here. For this reason, Dieterici, one of the most knowledgeable authorities on early consumption statistics, made the following statement:

situation of Germany around 1800 before the beginning of industrialization: low per capita real incomes and low consumption of animal proteins. Vegetable proteins will feed many more people more quickly than animal proteins.

The changes that have occurred over the last 150 or 100 years become even clearer if we make use of present-day nutritional units. Proteins, fats, carbohydrates, trace elements, and vitamins that cover the essential needs for growth and energy of the human organism can be obtained, in principle, from a wide variety of foodstuffs, depending on natural or man-made circumstances. Generally speaking, it can be estimated that the intake of energy-producing foods has steadily risen in the course of the nineteenth century. Since the turn of the century, that is, since the beginning of advanced industrialization in Germany, the level of intake per capita per year has remained more or less constant. Thereafter, food became increasingly refined, more digestible, and more varied—a process that was helped by some great inventions in food processing[11]—but the optimum quantitative level of consumption had already been

> It will prove impossible to give even an approximate quantitative description of many of these products; exact indications are available only for wine, tobacco, and sugar beets, since their production is subject to a tax. For almost all other cultivated plants, indications are not available, and for some of them, they do not even exist. Cabbage, vegetables, legumes, and rape cannot be measured statistically, since farmers cultivate them according to a variable demand. Carl Friedrich Wilhelm Dieterici, "Über die Verzehrung von Brod und Fleisch im Preussischen Staate," *Mittheilungen des statistischen Buros in Berlin,* 7 (1854): 135–152.

As long as we know nothing about the consumption of fruit and vegetables between 1800 and 1850, such rates of increase must be regarded with considerable caution. It is quite possible that consumption fell because of migration to the cities and the elimination of home garden production, but rose again later. However, it seems certain that the lower classes of the population ate very little fruit and vegetables by present-day standards, so that there still was an upward trend in consumption. In this connection, see also A. Hanau, "Entwicklungstendenzen der Ernährung in marktwirtschaftlicher Sicht," *Entwicklungstendenzen der Ernährung,* published by Forschungsrat für Ernährung, Landwirtschaft und Forsten (n.p., 1962).

11. In view of the latest inventions in the development of food for astronauts, artificial meat, food made from algae, diet foods, and vitaminization, the traditional view that all inventions in the field of food processing have already been made, and that henceforth the processing of food will only continue to use or simulate procedures of past epochs, no longer applies.

reached. It is an interesting fact that new developments in nutritional physiology and new techniques of food processing have since led to tendencies that have slowed down or even reversed the general trends outlined here. While the decreased consumption of vegetable fats in favor of animal proteins is without doubt characteristic of rising real incomes and industrialization, the decrease in Germany in the use of animal fats and butter in favor of certain highly refined vegetable fats (oil, vitaminized margarine, and so on) is an obvious fact. It almost seems that in this instance a secular trend has already passed its crest.

All of this is no doubt related to the already mentioned omnivorous constitution of man, who, when free to choose, desires a healthy, mixed diet. The study of historical changes in the intake of various nutritional elements should include the investigation in more depth of why certain foods were substituted for others and whether such substitutions entailed dislocations in physiological balance. Some of these shifts were particularly noteworthy. It seems, for example, that the decrease in carbohydrates from grain was at least partially compensated by an increase in carbohydrates from sugar. It is a well-known fact that in the eighteenth and especially in the early nineteenth century the potato (just like rice in many present-day developing countries) saved many people from starvation because of its high content in starch and vitamin C. These calories were later replaced by an increased consumption of fat, while increased consumption of tropical fruits (oranges and lemons) yielded the vitamin C. The place of legumes as a source of protein was taken by meat, fish, milk, cheese, and eggs. The place of whole-grain bread as the main source of protein, vitamin B_1, and calcium was later taken by fats, pork, milk, and cheese. White bread and rolls are satisfying and digestible, and their calories are easily assimilated, so that the great retreat of black bread in the nineteenth century is no historical accident.[12]

All of these dominating trends are relatively easily explained from a physiological and hygienic point of view. However—and

---

12. Glatzel, *Altbekanntes*.

this is the real starting point for any well-conceived history of nutrition—they were always limited by regional and social differences of income. Only those social groups that were economically somewhat better off were able to participate in the great shift toward a more refined and more rational diet in the first phase of industrialization. At the end of the nineteenth century, large segments of the lowest social classes did indeed eat less cereals, potatoes, legumes, flour products, and vegetable fats than at the beginning of the century, but they did not eat enough meat, butter, milk, cheese, eggs, sugar, fruit, and vegetables to overcome their earlier state of chronic malnutrition —for that is what we must call it from a modern vantage point—completely and everywhere. For the economically weak classes, the improvement consisted at first mainly in the changeover from a rough rural diet of markedly local character to a diet that quantitatively imitated upper-class food but failed to measure up to it in quality and therefore frequently had to make do with cheaper surrogates of the better foods and luxury items. The positive aspects of the ensuing refinement in the traditional vegetable diet, the introduction of new spices and luxuries for the broad masses, improvements in food processing and preparation, should not be overlooked. But despite all these improvements in the standard of nutrition, some profound differences in nutritional habits continued to exist for some time. As we suggested already, diet has always been subject to a number of natural, economic, technological, social, and cultural factors. The lucky "haves" have always enjoyed a better, more varied diet than their less fortunate contemporaries. But in earlier centuries, the procuring and preparation of food was largely regulated by tradition and station in life. People ate according to their estate, into which they were born just as they were born to a nationality. Just as it hardly ever occurred to the individual to break out of his station in life, so he could not conceive of changing the dietary habits befitting him. The seigneur ate in his castle and the day laborer ate in his cottage. The land brought forth all that was necessary, but any extensive trade in foodstuffs was unknown. Bad harvest and famines, like the great epidemics, were considered as periodically recurring natural disasters and simply had to be endured as sent by God. Good harvests brought lower food prices, bad harvests brought high prices and hard times to those who were not in a position to profit from high agricultural prices. With respect to food and drink, people lived more or less from hand to mouth; waste and gluttony abruptly gave way to equally extreme deprivation. The scenes of those great "pleasures of the table" as depicted, for example, in paintings by Pieter Brueghel the Elder or Rubens therefore do not tell us much about the secular trends in the standard of nutrition, quite aside from the fact that only well-to-do groups are portrayed. The land had to support only a relatively small population that reduced itself by emigration whenever there was a threat of overpopulation. By and large, no one thought that improvements in diet were needed, since people had very modest aspirations. Most of them tended to accept things as they found them. Only the nineteenth century saw a fundamental breakdown of the limitations imposed in nutritional habits by considerations of religion or estate. It was only now, for the first time in history, that nutrition became a problem that had to be studied and dealt with.

It is true that most people initially did not have the financial means to implement this emancipation and to adopt the dietary habits of the upper classes fully, and it is also true that customary norms in this area persisted for some time; nonetheless, the average person was systematically made aware of the inadequacy of his diet. Industrial society with its new needs and its decisive social dislocations—the key word "urbanization" immediately comes to mind—suddenly made the diet of the masses a problem that definitely became a part of the "social question." For the first time in human history, food no longer was simply grown where people lived, but had to be planned for in some unified fashion and purchased with money. It is no accident that the period of industrial mass nutrition in the nineteenth century marks the beginning of the scientific investigation of standards of living, household budgets, and the nutritional requirements of man. Science discovered how many factors influence the energy and the regenerative powers of a working human being; and even the state realized, for example, that a well-nourished work force is much more productive for the nation than a malnourished one. Within a few decades, an almost dramatic change occurred in the age-old and rather remarkably stable and uniform nutritional habits that had proved inappropriate and insufficient. This much, then, for a short survey of the secular tendencies in the changing standards of nutrition.

The Elimination of Periodic Famines

A more detailed survey, showing the individual highs and lows of food supply, reveals that the entire eighteenth and also the first half of the nineteenth century showed signs of specific shortages that no longer exist in Germany today. The potato blight of 1843 and 1845, for example, brought serious nutritional crises leading to hunger typhus and other epidemics that are attested to by well-known contemporary accounts. Without belittling the extent of the suffering in any way, it must be said that these hunger catastrophes should be seen in comparison with the periodic famines of the Middle Ages, the Thirty Years' War, and even the eighteenth century. Comparative data are not yet available, but the findings of the newest research permit us to assume that the starving Silesian weavers were not nearly as desperate as people caught up in earlier famines or even the starving populations of present-day India or Biafra. In any case, there are no accounts of cannibalism for the hunger periods of the 1840s, while we hear of it again and again from the Middle Ages into the seventeenth century. It would certainly be quite wrong to paint an idyllic picture of the nutrition of the lower classes in pre-industrial times. As we have already pointed out, the greatest abundance of food and stark misery often existed almost side by side, but because of the lack of communication, it was often impossible to distribute supplies. A rapid glance at the older literature shows that earlier foods crises were much more extensive. According to the chronicles of Mark-Brandenburg, there were serious famines in 1312, 1352, 1362, 1397, 1416, 1426, 1467, and 1527.[13] We are told that in 1548 people took grain from the fields and roasted it before it was ripe. A history of the town of Spandau relates that in 1598 1,000 of the 3 or 4,000 inhabitants died from a pestilent disease caused by hunger. Johann Crüvel's *Kremmenscher Schau-Bühne* reports that the years 1637–39 witnessed great misery after the harvest had failed completely. The country people and the soldiers ate cats, mice, dead animals, as well as their fellow men. There were mobs before the gates of the town of Brandenburg demanding the putrifying carcasses of animals. In Wittenberg, lots were cast to determine who should die first in order to be eaten. Even those who had money could not buy grain. One officer relates that some poor, starving people ran toward him and asked him to give them the dog with him so that they might eat it. Feeling sorry for them, he offered them money, but they did not want it, since it would not buy them food. He gave them the dog. Such accounts are frequently found in writings from the late Middle Ages to the nineteenth century. If the weavers' revolt in Silesia and the hunger crises of those days [the 1840s] are still remembered as social calamities of the first order, this fact is probably related to the extensive public discussion that took place in the context of the emerging "social question." This was the time when the literature about pauperism was able to grow by leaps and bounds following the relaxation of censorship. There was a new awareness of the misery of the lower classes and of the special situation of wage labor; everyone was talking and writing about it. By comparison, the contemporary writing during earlier hunger crises, such as the famine of 1770 or the agrarian crises of the early nineteenth century with the three phases 1801–05, 1806–17, and 1818–30 is surprisingly scanty. Obviously,

---

13. These dates are taken from F. S. Bock, *Versuch einer wirtschaftlichen Naturgeschichte von dem Königreich Ost-und Westpreussen*, 5 vols. (Dessau, 1782). For the problem of famines, cf. also Friedrich Curschmann, *Hungersnöte im Mittelalter* (Leipzig, 1900); Karl Biedermann, *Deutschland im 18. Jahrhundert*, 2 vols. (Leipzig, 1854–58); Abel, *Agrarkrisen*.

hunger was still considered a blow of fortune and there was little point in writing about it. Yet these earlier crises must have been much more acute, if only because money was no remedy, since trade and communication, which might have equalized the situation, were nonexistent. Nor was it easy, until the nineteenth century, to switch to the potato when grain failed. There is no longer any doubt that the potato, once it was established as a standard food item for human consumption, helped to prevent the worst. Furthermore, the abolition of the strict three-field system made it possible to cultivate turnips, maize, carrots, and other crops temporarily on a large scale. In addition, turnips and clover partly took the place of the grain that had hitherto been used as feed for livestock. The Prussian statistician Dieterici reported that earlier centuries were characterized not only by periodic famines, but also by frequent shortages.[14] On the basis of the chronicles studied, he estimated that, in a single German principality, such minor crises occurred on the average of one every four or five years. Furthermore, fluctuations of price were much greater then than in the nineteenth century. For, as Adam Smith observed, English grain prices as late as in the seventeenth and eighteenth century varied on a scale of 1 to 5, and according to the English statistician Bowring, the prices of grain for export to Danzig and Königsberg in the late eighteenth century varied on scale of 1 to 4 over relatively short periods. In the eighteenth century, grain prices in Berlin showed differences of 1 to 3.5, while by the middle of the nineteenth century, we hear complaints about differences of only 1 to 2 and 1 to 1.25. In contrast with earlier centuries, some aid already flowed into the affected areas during the great Silesian famine of 1846–47, and charities were founded in cities everywhere, so that a number of relief measures could be taken whenever there was a rise in the price of grain or potatoes. By the nineteenth century, charitable institutions had broken out of a strictly local framework. This fact too marks a change from the nutritional situation of earlier centuries.

14. Dieterici, "Über die Verzehrung."

The drastic improvement in the nutritional situation of Germany is illustrated by a comparison of menus from North German poorhouses between 1785 and 1849 with the diet in similar mass kitchens around 1900 and again in 1967.[15] These menus indicate that in the late eighteenth century the inmates of poorhouses lived mainly on cereals and legumes, and around 1840 usually on potatoes. By 1900, however, their diet had improved to an almost incredible degree, as is also shown by detailed household budgets of worker families in Frankfurt, Mannheim, and Switzerland. By present-day standards, the diet of the lower classes around 1900 was still quite rudimentary and monotonous, but by comparison with 1785 and 1840 it had improved enormously in quantity and quality. . . . An analysis of these menus illustrates once again that the social critics of the late nineteenth century were very much mistaken when they charged their own time with responsibility for all social evils. To this day, there is a certain historical school of thought that ascribes all of the misery of the lower social classes to industrialization and sees a progressive deterioration in the standard of living of the broad masses due to the expansion of capitalism. But the available facts do not bear out such theories. The fact is that Germany, like the other industrial states of Western and Central Europe, was no longer subject to real famines once the transition to more advanced forms of technology and economy had been completed under the impact of industrialization. As Wilhelm Abel . . . has rightly said, it is very difficult to establish precisely when the secular low point in the food supply of Central Europe was definitely overcome, since short-term oscillations in the price and wage structure disguise the long-term trends of the century. Nonetheless, it seems clear that a safe margin of food supply and a fundamental improvement in the standard of nutrition were achieved by the middle of the nineteenth century.

An important indicator for this fact is, once again, the consumption of meat. According to Table 16 of the present study

15. Abel, *Agrarkrisen*, p. 237.

[omitted here], meat consumption per person per year in the area of the future German Empire amounted to only 13.7 kg. in the years after the Napoleonic Wars, which coincided with extensive crop failures and local famines in 1816–17. It appears that this annual consumption, despite sporadic declines, had risen very slightly by the third phase (1818–30) of the agrarian crisis. Following the statistics, we see a period of relative stagnation between 1830 and 1850. The decisive breakthrough occurred in the middle of the 1850s. By 1871, the annual per capita consumption was 29.4 kg.; in 1892, it amounted to 39.3 kg.; and by 1910 it had reached 46.7 kg.

The definitive establishment of a safe margin of food supply and the improvement in the standard of nutrition were achieved mainly by three factors:

1. By the agricultural revolution, that is, an unprecedented rise in productivity brought about by a new system of crop rotation, the introduction of artificial fertilizers and mechanization, as well as by a new distribution of the land following agrarian-reform legislation.

2. By the transportation revolution—in this case the possibility of using transatlantic shipping and the railroads for the large-scale transport of foodstuffs. (From about 1850, the agrarian countries overseas and in Eastern Europe were increasingly able to fill gaps in the food supply with their surplus grain and meat whenever it became necessary, to the point where cheap American grain caused a collapse of grain prices in Germany, an agrarian crisis, and the establishment of protective tariffs.)

3. By the revolutionary new methods of food preservation in the pre-industrial period that for the first time in history made it possible to keep and transport foodstuffs for prolonged periods without impairing their flavor or quality.

From this time on, Germany has become virtually immune to the consequences of crop failures. Subsequent food crises were no longer famines, but were characterized by high food prices. The idea that food itself might become scarce has disappeared from public consciousness with amazing rapidity. "Give us this day our daily bread," that age-old biblical prayer, in response to a concrete need, was applied (to state it with some exaggeration) to a minor, remediable mishap in a highly mechanized food industry or in an increasingly efficient welfare state. The steady stream of imports from overseas and the new methods of food preservation also lessened the impact of seasonal changes. Fresh meat, traditionally available only during a few months of the year, now was in constant supply throughout the year. All this is part of the extraordinary evolution in the eighteenth and nineteenth century that Werner Sombart characterized with the felicitous term "emancipation from the bonds of nature."

The New Function of Money in Providing Food

Industrialization has restructured the standard of nutrition in Germany in several important ways. First, the daily necessities of life were no longer received in kind, but through the intermediary of money. As the Swiss scholar R. Braun has pointed out, the importance of the introduction of this exogenous medium into daily life can hardly be exaggerated in its consequences for the change in nutritional habits. The population was split, as it were, into two antagonistic parts, one landless and one landowning; and this fact was at least as decisive for the formation of social classes as the ownership or nonownership of the means of production. That part of the "working classes" that left the land, and consequently all domestic production of food, was henceforth obliged to purchase all food by means of money, a situation that had always been considered exceptional in the traditional agrarian society—to use in this case this rather vague model. It is true that ever since the older seigneuries were rented out, some of the feudal tenants [*Hörige*] paid their landlords in money, but this money was practically never used to buy food staples. In the relatively thinly populated towns as well, people consumed a "peasant diet," raising much of their food themselves. Thus Goethe tells us that in Heilbronn the owners of small houses still used the streets and alleys along the town walls away from the main street for depositing manure. In 1786, the town of Hanover, one of the largest capitals of Germany, with 20,000 inhabitants, still counted 365 head of cattle within its walls.[16] While it is true that the wage earner who was no longer paid in kind became increasingly dependent on money, it is also true that he was able to exercise much greater freedom in the choice of his food and to expand the range of the foods he consumed to a considerable extent. The emancipation from a rather monotonous local and regional diet and from the strictures of a social or religious nature, the adoption of entirely new criteria in the choice of food, and the stimulation of new desires by advertising have considerably lessened the differences in taste between the lower and the privileged upper classes, leading to the beginning of something that might be called the "democratization of dietary gratification." At the same time, all these developments also had their effect on agricultural production and in turn contributed to its commercialization. The fact that the decline of traditional food habits was accompanied by an expanded range of financially accessible foodstuffs and —at least to some degree—slowly brought the lower classes into contact with new food items must be considered one of the most far-reaching results of this evolution. Another aspect of the new structure of daily eating and drinking was the fact that the new class of pure consumers became dependent on the increasing number of grocers, who, significantly, were originally called *Kolonialwarenhändler* [literally, dealers in colonial, or tropical, products] in Germany. The founding of workers' consumer cooperatives, soup kitchens, factory canteens, workers' restaurants, cooperative kitchens, dairies, and coffee houses, and even of *Schrebergärten** clubs can also be interpreted as attempts to mitigate the disadvantage of this dependence. The barter system—that is, the payment of factory workers in merchandise

---

*Schrebergärten are rented plots of land, usually at the edge of the city, where apartment-dwellers raise fruit and vegetables.–Trans.

16. Georg von Viehbahn, *Statistik des zollvereinten und nördlichen Deutschlands*, vol. 2 (Berlin, 1862), p. 860. In 1891, Oetker's invention of baking powder, following some earlier experiments in this direction by Liebig, led to a major change in commercial and domestic baking. Cf. Franz Lerner, *Handel, Hausfrau und Hausbäckerei*, pamphlet distributed by Dr. August Oetker GmbH (Bielefeld, 1956).

rather than money—a phenomenon that, according to the latest research, was related in part to an insufficient circulation of specie in the early stages of industrialization, is germane to this problem. However, this process of commercialization of food, which led to extremely unfortunate social abuses in the early stages of industrialization, was by and large a fact of the last third of the nineteenth century and must not be overstated for the beginning of the century. As late as 1860, for example, two-thirds of all the bread consumed in Germany was still baked in private homes according to reliable contemporary statistics.[17] Even in industrial areas, the workers, especially those working at home, often held on to a small plot of land for a long time, so that the process of commercialization of food really moved into full gear only with the foundation of Bismarck's empire. It was only when the workers moved into the large tenement houses following the East-West migration that money began to play a dominant role in the daily acquisition of food. Up to 1870, most Germans lived in the country or in small towns and therefore usually consumed only what they produced themselves.[18]

It is remarkable that the emerging workers' movement was already aware of this far-reaching structural change in the ordinary conduct of the household. In his widely read book *Die Frau und der Sozialismus (Woman and Socialism)* (1883), August Bebel expressed the opinion that for millions of women the individual kitchen is "one of the most exhausting, time-consuming, and wasteful institutions, which ruins their health and their disposition." He felt that doing away once and for all with individual cooking would be a blessing for countless women. In the socialist society he envisaged, there were to be only mass kitchens, which, being equipped in the most modern way, would prepare food much more economically than a proliferation of

17. Rudolf Heberle, *Die Grosstädte im Strom der Binnenwanderung* (Leipzig, 1937); Wilhelm Brepohl, *Der Aufbau des Ruhrvolkes im Zuge der Ost-Westwanderung* (Recklinghausen, 1948); W. Brepohl, *Industrievolk im Wandel von der agraren zur industriellen Daseinsform* (Tübingen, 1957); Lothar Schneider, *Der Arbeiterhaushalt im 18. und 19. Jahrhundert: Dargestellt am Beispiel des Heim- und Fabrikarbeiters* (Berlin, 1967).

18. Willy Hellpach, *Mensch und Volk in der Grosstadt*, 2nd ed. (Stuttgart, 1952).

private households. In order to avoid the new consumer dependence created by a capitalist economy, the great socialist leader wanted to establish a system of food preparation that was totally collective as well as scientific and efficient. In the same book, Bebel also proposed a qualitative change in diet. He pointed out that large segments of the German population still lived mainly on potatoes, unable to afford meat. The socialist society he envisioned would therefore have to see to it that a sufficient quantity of meat was available to everyone. At the same time, he stressed the importance of vegetables, which would have to be raised on a large scale. Furthermore, chemistry "would henceforth deploy an unprecedented activity in the production of new and improved foods." Thus the workers' movement had not remained untouched by developments in the nascent science of nutrition and anticipated a "total revolution of domestic life."

The Effects of Factory Work on Meals

It is well known that factory work has caused the greatest dislocation in the diet of the lower social classes. Fixed working hours that sharply divided the working person's day into work and free time, separate places for working and living due to the increasingly centralized process of production, and finally man's adaptation to the machine and its new rhythm decisively altered the dietary habits of the world of agriculture and the traditional trades. Henceforth, eating and drinking served not only to appease feelings of hunger and thirst, but also, among other things, to provide an interruption in a monotonous workday of ten, twelve, or more hours. As the reports of factory inspectors show, inexpensive stimulants were increasingly used to "kill time." The drinking of coffee was particularly important for cottage workers. It was one of the inconveniences of factory work that breakfast had to be taken very early in the morning or hastily during working hours, since most factory regulations provided for only one break at noon. The breakfast break was, and remained for a long time, the privilege of the foreman in the factory. If the wife worked in the factory too, the noon break was hardly sufficient for the preparation of a meal; as a result, the food was often half-done and poorly prepared. If the worker's home was too far away, the noon meal was taken outdoors or on the job. The machine no longer permitted the "luxury" of a long interruption for eating. While, in the early stages of industrialization in Germany, it was possible to spend as much as two hours for a meal, as is still the custom in certain Mediterranean countries, the time spent for meals in the industrial age had to be strictly curtailed and, as it were, adapted to the requirements of the machine age. Factory inspectors tell us again and again that a piece of sausage, a slab of boiled bacon, and a sip from the brandy flask (sometimes called *Flachmann*, since its flat shape made it easy to carry in one's pocket) had to serve as breakfast and lunch for the urban industrial worker, a fact that immediately explains the intense preoccupation with the problem of alcohol in these reports.

In 1885, the factor inspector, Fridolin Schuler, described the nutritional situation of the worker families he had visited as follows:

> Traditionally, the housewife remained at home. She left home only to work in the field, and if for some reason she occasionally did not have time to cook a proper meal, older girls would take her place in the kitchen. Nowadays, the entire family works in the factory. In the morning, the wife must get to the kitchen very early—one of the children may have to report to the factory, a half hour away, by six o'clock even in the winter—so breakfast has to be fixed in a hurry. A half hour before the noon meal, the mother leaves her job in the factory, rushes home, and cooks as quickly as possible, for soon the family will be home to eat and will complain if the steaming bowl is not already on the table. An hour later, the whole family will be back on the job in the factory. Where can she find time for any proper cooking and where will her daughter learn to cook if she is constantly working in the factory?[19]

---

19. Fridolin Schuler, "Die glarnerische Baumwollindustrie und ihr Einfluss auf die Gesundheit der Arbeiter," *Zeitschrift für Schweizerische Statistik*, 1872, pp. 215–216.

According to Schuler's observations, in this case referring to the textile industry in the upper part of the Zurich canton, the worker's table was in poor shape indeed. In the morning, the meal usually consisted of potato hash, taken with a great deal of chicory coffee that contained a few real coffee beans and some milk. The children ate the same food. At noon, since time was short, there was more of the same coffee as well as buttered bread and cheese; on a good day, there might be a flour or potato soup with quick-cooked vegetables. These Swiss working-class families, like those in southern Germany, consumed a great deal of baked or cooked pastry, but in Schuler's opinion, it was ruined by the lack of baking and cooking skill of the "factory women." They would quickly knead together a simple dough that was rapidly baked at excessive temperatures in order to have the meal ready as soon as possible. Thus the family was often served a dish that was undone on the inside and burned on the outside. And as the food deteriorated, the temptation of alcohol became greater. Cheap liquor had to make up for inadequate food. In this manner, many a family became caught in a dreadful vicious cycle: The lack of work opportunities in the countryside forced entire families to work in the newly established factories in the cities. Now almost full-time absence of the wife and her older daughter from home brought a deterioration of the food eaten by the whole family. This in turn led to an increased consumption of liquor. The ensuing malnutrition and alcoholism finally led to reduced income, loss of job, or premature invalidity. Eventually a way out of this vicious cycle was provided by rising real wages, decline of woman and child labor, and an increased number of factory canteens.

Nevertheless, the aftereffects of this dreadful situation persisted for a long time. A German miner who had worked for some time in England at the end of the nineteenth century painted the following picture of English working-class women:

> The English workers' wives are often incapable of fixing a meal, but what they do know is whiskey drinking. I have seen things that you wouldn't believe in Germany. . . . It is a sure thing that more women are taken with drink than men. The factory workers'

wives are usually drunks. What this does to morality can easily be imagined. Married women offer themselves when they are drunk. . . . One of the reasons is probably that the women can't find work. . . . These women are too lazy to sew, even though all girls have to learn sewing in school. A foreigner who doesn't know the situation will be shocked if he walks through the working-class neighborhood around nine or ten in the morning and sees that two-thirds of the women have simply pinned their clothes together instead of sewing them, and that they are neither combed nor washed.[20]

The Swedish social critic Gustav Steffen reported that the women in the English textile town of Oldham (near Manchester) were all indifferent or poor housekeepers who would rather buy expensive, unnecessarily refined food than learn to cook properly. If at the end of the week they were short of money, the family's food became much worse than it needed to be. These people ate canned meat, fish, vegetables, fruit, and even milk and used egg powder instead of eggs, soup extract from tin cans instead of real soup.

The effects of factory work also reached down into the profoundest depths of the human psyche by secularizing or even rendering obsolete solemn prescriptions and injunctions of cultic and magic origin that had, in time, been cast in religious terms. As we know, eating and drinking had been dissociated from their function of satisfying hunger and thirst in the earliest stages of civilization and were subjected to strict codes of behavior that evolved into very complex systems with sometimes rather draconian rules. Many of these rules persist to this day, despite all change, as simple conventions: for example, the custom of drinking to someone's health, the use of knife and fork for specific dishes, the sequence of courses and beverages. The simple fact that the urban industrial worker took at least two of his daily meals no longer with his family, as people had done for thousands of years, but more or less alone among other workers at his place of work, and under the pressure of time, was bound

20. E. Dückershof, *Wie lebt der englische Arbeiter?* (Dresden, 1898), pp. 19, 32–33.

to change the very concept of eating in the most fundamental way. Above all, the almost complete destruction of the family's *communio epulandi et potandi*, that regular structure of common meals with its originally cultic and magic, later religious, connotations (recall that even today baptisms, weddings, funerals, and confirmations are occasions for communal meals) had far-reaching consequences.[21] This is an essential but unfortunately rather unexplored aspect of the process of separation between living and working space during industrialization, and the sociology of work and industry is still trying to assess its effects.

On the other hand, this process of making food intake "efficient" in a secular sense also led to the elaboration of new rules of behavior. In keeping with Ludwig Feuerbach's materialist maxim, "Man is what he eats," people often ate as much as they "could afford" in the second half of the nineteenth century, as the standard of living was generally improving by comparison with the periodic famines and shortages of the preceding centuries. At times, the *embonpoint* was considered a mark of social prestige, setting its owner apart from the "starving wretches." The old legend of alcohol as well, namely, the idea that the ability to drink great quantities is a mark of virility, received new impetus. Gluttony and immoderate drinking, both of which are undoubtedly related to the age-old fallacy that it is possible to acquire special powers, talents, and faculties by ingesting certain solid or liquid substances (compare the practice of blood brotherhood) have, of course, always existed, but it was only the industrial age that made them into social criteria within the working classes. By the turn of the century, the beginnings of the science of nutrition first caused women to worry about their figures; at the same time vegetarianism, uncooked foods, whole grains, *Kneipp* diets, Bircher's *muesli*, and so on, became the fashion. The sudden rash of writings against "inelegant" corpulence and for a "healthy, natural way of life" around 1900 almost seismographically shows this change in the standard of nutrition.

21. Hellpach, *Mensch und Volk in der Grosstadt*.

Exclusively sedentary or standing work in closed, frequently overheated, poorly ventilated, or dust-filled rooms; a decrease in heavy physical work and an increasing need for mental concentration, quick reaction, and adaptability; the adoption of a completely new daily rhythm of life and work; the loss of traditional domestic production and the resulting dependence on the constant fluctuations of the market; the shift from the extended rural family with its patriarchic, traditionally religious ways to the secularized, money-and-achievement-oriented nuclear family with its higher expectations—these and other factors have contributed to a qualitative change in the standard of nutrition. By the end of the nineteenth century, the household was certainly not yet what we know it to be today, but it did have more in common with the present-day household than with that of the middle of the eighteenth century. Meat, cold cuts, chicory coffee, sugar, and brandy had become part of the diet of the lower classes by the end of the nineteenth century. By comparison with the period around 1800, the urban industrial worker preferred lighter, more nutritious, more digestible foods that not only "stuck to his ribs," but also were more stimulating to the sense of taste and smell. The generally increased intake of animal proteins also permitted longer uninterrupted periods of work. "Second breakfast" and "afternoon coffee" were still a regular and widespread feature of the daily meal plan for cottage workers in the first half of the nineteenth century, but these supplementary meals became increasingly rare as the century drew to a close. All of this should be interpreted as a sign of increased individual productivity and an adaptation to the requirements of the modern industrial world.

The Beginning of the Age of Canned Food

It is no accident that the beginning of the "age of canned food"—or more precisely, the age of increased demand for pre-prepared foods in concentrated form that can be stored for prolonged periods of time without appreciable loss of flavor and nutritional value, and can be prepared rapidly without much competence in cooking—coincided with the beginning of industrialization. Unfortunately, neither the history of the techniques of food preservation nor the history of the industries engaged in canning or the manufacture of macaroni products, jams, and soup concentrates has so far been written in sufficient depth or breadth. It is therefore necessary to piece together this information from widely scattered monographs.[22] Yet this is a central chapter in the development of the standard of nutrition in Germany in the nineteenth century. Nowhere can we study the influence of the industrializing economy on the nutritional habits of the population better than here.

The various techniques of keeping, storing, and even "preserving" foods and beverages as a protection against fermentation, spoilage, and putrefaction are, of course, as old as the conscious management of food itself and, like cooking, must be counted among the oldest techniques of human civilization. For thousands of years, these techniques of preservation had been limited to cooking, salting, drying, smoking, baking, and fermenting in the individual household and exclusively for home consumption. Only a very few sectors had developed a trade to handle such production—for example, the drying of fruit. However, the commercially available foods that could be kept for a limited time played practically no role at all in the nutrition of

22. Cf., for example, B. Winkler, "Aus der Geschichte der Obst- und Gemüseverwertungsindustrie in Deutschland," *Industrielle Obst- und Gemüseverwertung, 1962* (Braunschweig, 1963); W. Herrmann, "Aus Vergangenheit und Gegenwart der deutschen Obst- und Gemüsekonservenindustrie," *Zeitschrift für handelswissenschaftliche Forschung* 3 (1951); J. Schorrmüller, *Lehrbuch der Lebensmittelchemie* (Berlin, Göttingen, and Heidelberg, 1961); Nehring-Krause, *Konserventechnisches Handbuch*, 15th ed., vol. 2 (Braunschweig, 1969); F. Grüttner, *Geschichte der Fleischversorgung in Deutschland* (Braunschweig, 1938); E. Bergdolt, "Die exportierende Fleischindustrie Nord- und Südamerikas seit 1913" (Ph.D. diss. Hamburg, 1924); H. Göben, *Die Fischwirtschaft in Zahlen* (Braunschweig, 1967); R. Hennig, *Fischwarenkunde*, 5th ed. (Leipzig, 1959); F. Lücke, *Fischindustrielles Taschenbuch*, 4th ed. (Braunschweig, 1954); K. Joachim, "Die Fleischversorgung der Provinz Hannover während der Zwangsbewirtschaftung von 1916 bis 1920" (Ph.D. diss., Hamburg, 1924). I am most obliged to Mr. Erhart Busche for his help in gathering and evaluating this scattered literature. Furthermore, my conversations with him generated a number of new ideas.

the broad masses. They were either luxury items for small privileged groups or else they were used as supplies for ship's crews, expeditions, or in special cases, armies. In this area, the nineteenth century developed revolutionary new methods, such as heating in a vacuum until sterilization, the use of new antiseptic preservatives (alcohol, highly concentrated sugar solutions, glycerin, volatile oils, salycilic, sulphuric, and benzoic acids), the beginning of freezing techniques in freezers of various kinds in conjunction with the use of salt solutions, and as a final treatment, electromagnetic current, as well as the use of new hermetically sealing covers. All these techniques were exploited by new industries, which increasingly displaced the traditional domestic practices.

By far the most frequently used and effective method was that of heating in a vacuum, which was discovered, independently it seems, and almost simultaneously, in France and England. As far as can be ascertained, the evolution began with the invention of the "digester" by Denis Papin in London in 1681. This kettle was made of bronze and had a tightly closing lid. Fitted with a safety valve, a pressure gauge, and a thermometer, it was filled with water and then heated. This led Papin to the discovery of the law of physics that pressure in a closed space increases with the rise of temperature. "Papin's digester," which is said to have been used for preserving foods, is thus not only a starting point for later pressure cookers and steam engines, but also for modern canning techniques.[23]

The personal cook of Duke Christian IV of Pfalz-Zweibrücken, Nicolas-François Appert (1750–1841), is said to have been the first to have made practical use of this invention, which is why the heating of food in a vacuum was at first called

---

23. Recall that Denis Papin (1647–1712) started out as a physician in Paris, then spent time as assistant to the famous scientist Boyle in London, and finally was professor of mathematics and physics in Marburg (1688–1704). While in Cornwall, Papin had probably become acquainted with Thomas Savary's steam engine, patented by the latter in 1698. Papin's digester was based on Savary's principle. Cf. E. Gerland, *Leibnizens und Huygens' Briefwechsel mit Papin nebst Biographie Papins* (Leipzig, 1881); Karl Karmarsch, *Geschichte der Technologie seit der Mitte des achtzehnten Jahrhunderts* (Munich, 1872), p. 118.

"appertizing." Appert, who later became a dealer in dainty pastries, a manufacturer of liqueurs, a writer about food, and a philanthropist, was praised in the *Courier d'Europe* of February 10, 1809, as the inventor of this method of preservation.[24] The article said enthusiastically that Appert had discovered the secret of arresting the seasons: spring, summer, and autumn would live on, as it were, in bottles. The article pointed to the extraordinary benefits of this invention for trade, medicine, navigation, armies, and colonies. The new methods would make it possible to cheer up a depressed patient in the middle of winter with fruit in its natural color and unadulterated flavor; at the same time, it would be possible to save half the sugar, a fact that seemed particularly attractive given the scarcity of that commodity due to the Continental System and the English blockade. In 1801, Napoleon I granted a prize of 12,000 gold fancs to the inventor, subject to the condition that he publish his invention for the benefit of all. This was done in the same year and Appert described his procedure as follows:

1. All substances to be preserved must be enclosed in *"bouteilles"* or other large glass containers.
2. These receptacles must be closed "with the utmost exactitude," since success depends, above all, on proper closing.
3. The substances enclosed in this manner must be exposed to the effects of boiling water in a water bath for a shorter or longer time, depending on the nature of the substance.
4. The receptacles must be removed from the water bath at the proper time.

According to some sources, Appert had experimented only with glass receptacles. After the Napoleonic Wars, when he wanted to turn to the commercial exploitation of his invention, he realized to his dismay that the English in particular were already widely using it and had even developed it further, independently of him. P. Durand, among others, had also realized

---

24. Nicholas-François Appert, *Die Kunst alle animalischen und vegetabilischen Substanzen mehrere Jahre zu erhalten*, trans. from the French (Vienna, 1832), pp. v ff.

the importance of sterilization during the boiling process and had been able, around 1810, to preserve foods in tin-plated cans.[25] For his part, Appert continued to receive the highest honors—he was given the title of "Benefactor of Humanity"—and constantly worked on related experiments. He experimented with the purification of fermented beverages, with concentrating new wine, and with heating wine for preservation, all of which, among other things, helped pave the way for Justus Liebig and Louis Pasteur. Nonetheless, Appert died almost penniless, having spent all his money on his experiments. In 1830, his son, François Appert, wrote a book explaining theoretically, for the first time, the process of preservation by means of heat in a vacuum; he also described the tin-plated can as the optimal receptacle. It is not certain, however, whether we should consider 1830 the beginning of the "age of the tin can," as some authors do, since the British fleet, especially the great East-Indiamen, had used pork in soldered tin cans, manufactured in a factory in Cork, Ireland, long before there was a theoretical explanation of the process.

Appert's writings had been translated into several languages shortly after the Napoleonic Wars. The shipping trade was particularly interested in canned goods, so that the techniques were rapidly perfected. In Germany, however, the traditional domestic methods of preservation continued to be used, since there was no market for the expensive canned goods. In 1840, the Frankfurt physician Georg Varrentrapp gave a lecture to the Society for the Advancement of Trade and Industry in Braunschweig in which he described the canning industry he had seen while traveling in England. Following his lecture, a few local tinsmiths attempted to make tin containers for preserving asparagus, but apparently it was done only for their own use or by special order.[26]

As far as we now know, the beginning of industrial canning in

---

25. Herrmann, *Obst- und Gemüsekonservenindustrie*, p. 245; Gustaf Steffen, *Streifzüge durch Grossbritannien* (Stuttgart, 1896), p. 125; Steffen, *England als Weltmacht und Kulturstaat* (Stuttgart, 1899), p. 223.

26. Georg Varrentrapp, *Tagebuch einer medizinischen Reise nach England, Holland und Belgien* (Frankfurt,/M. 1839); Herrmann, *Obst- und Gemüsekonservenindustrie*, p. 246.

RELATIONSHIP BETWEEN DIET AND INDUSTRIALIZATION

Germany was marked by the first attempts of the firms Daniel Heinrich Carstens in Lübeck (1845) and Bethmann Brothers in Frankfurt-am-Main (1845). Shortly thereafter, two Braunschweig tinsmiths, Pillmann (1850) and Daubert (1860), preserved asparagus, beans, and peas in cans.[27] Altogether, however, this production probably amounted to only a few thousand cans per year.[28] Although Appert had already preserved virtually all kinds of foods in his bottles and glass jars (vegetables, fruits, meat, fish, butter, milk, beer, coffee, broth, even "pre-prepared dishes"), industrial production was initially limited almost entirely to vegetables. It was only in the 1850s that commercial canning of fruit was started in California and, shortly thereafter, that of dairy products in Switzerland. During the Crimean War (1853–56) the Anglo-French forces used canned foods for their troops on a large scale for the first time, although the English navy, as we pointed out, had made use of them earlier. Within a few decades, industrially preserved foods now became standard equipment for active military service. Following the example of the adversary, the German General Staff became convinced of the usefulness of canning during the War of 1870–71. Since it was known that during the American Civil War (1861–65) a great deal of food adulteration had been perpetrated, especially in canned goods, the German government founded its own factories, which, among other things, manufactured the famous *Erbswurst*. The latter was an invention of the cook Grüneberg of Berlin (d. 1872) and consisted of a mixture of dried pea meal, bacon, and spices tightly packed in a casing of waxed paper. Every German soldier on his way to the front has carried it in his knapsack ever since. It was part of the famous "iron ration" and could be counted on to produce a substantial meal quickly, by the simple expedient of dissolving it in water and bringing the mixture to a boil.

Another boon to the developing food industry was the invention of meat extract by two Frenchmen, Proust and Parmentier. After 1830, meat bouillon was boiled down to a thick soup. In

---

27. Winkler, *Geschichte der Obst- und Gemüseverwertungsindustrie*, p. 258.
28. Herrmann, *Obst- und Gemüsekonservenindustrie*.

dried form, these "bouillon bars" were used as rations on ships and also sold as strengthening medicines in pharmacies. Large-scale production of meat extract became possible only when, in 1857, Liebig invented an efficient method of obtaining "extractum carnis" in the context of his research on the constituent parts of muscle meat, and his pupil, the Munich physician and pharmacist Max Pettenkofer (1818–1901), conducted the necessary experiments for the practical application of these ideas. Large meat factories were built in Fray Bentos, Uruguay, where after 1864 the meat of 150,000 to 200,000 cattle per year was processed. After all the fat was cut off, the meat was boiled down to a brown powder, which, packed in cans, kept extremely well and could easily be shipped over long distances, even halfway around the world. Suddenly the great herds of cattle in Argentina, North America, New Zealand, and Australia became very important to the European market. The techniques of preservation created entirely new configurations in the world economy and stimulated international trade in an unprecedented way. In Germany, "Liebig's meat extract" became a popular condiment and gave rise to an entire industry engaged in the manufacture of bouillon cubes and dried soups. A specialized cookbook on the use of the new industrial consommés was published as early as 1870.[29]

Beginning in the 1850s and rapidly multiplying in the 1880s, meat and meat-product factories were initially the most important branch of the developing food industry. This rapid industrialization of meat production was related to the discovery of the trichina worm and to the introduction of official meat inspection, to the establishment of municipal slaughterhouses (10 for all of Prussia in 1880, 180 in 1890, and 500 in 1908), but also to revolutionary improvements in the techniques of refrigeration and transportation.[30] In 1896, after some initial failures, the

---

29. Henriette Davidis, *Kraftbrühe aus Liebigs Fleischextrakt* (Braunschweig, 1870).

30. Ostertag, *Handbuch der Fleischbeschau und Leitfaden für Fleischbeschauer*, 2 vols., 8th ed. (Berlin, 1922–23); Schlampp, *Die Fleischgesetzgebung in sämtlichen Bundesstaaten* (Berlin, 1892); Emmerich Reek, *Die Frankfurter Würstchen*, ed. F. Lerner, (Frankfurt,/M. 1939).

canned frankfurter conquered the market of modest restaurants and the public in general. The first frankfurter cannery had been opened by the butcher Heine of Halberstadt the year before. Some butchers in Braunschweig and Frankfurt-am-Main soon followed his example. The great success of canned meat was due, among other things, to the fact that the products could be mildly cured, thus yielding a much more delicate flavor than traditional dried and salted meats could achieve. Especially for the perishable frankfurter sausage, the hermetically sealed tin can was an ideal container. Soon the "frank" in its new container made its way around the world. But since slaughtering now took place throughout the year, since the slaughterhouses were never too distant from the grazing grounds, and since, in any case, the transport of living meat-cattle was not too expensive, fresh meat continued to dominate the market in the German towns. There was no need to preserve meat, so that there was a built-in ceiling on the production of canned meat. World War I, however, brought an abrupt rise in the demand for canned meat. The army established meat-canning factories in Spandau and Mainz, which produced 8 million cans per month in shifts around the clock.[31] In 1918, some 11,000 persons were engaged in the production of canned goods for the army alone. Under the system of state control during the war, many municipalities collected large stores of meat during the summer months and had to build special refrigerating facilities for them. This "frozen meat" eventually became the main competitor for canned meat. In general, however, production in Germany remained far below the United States, where in 1920 the largest meat processors (the Big Five) employed some 50,000 persons, processing 300,000 hogs, 95,000 cattle, and 180,000 sheep per week and producing 500,000 cans per day.

The rise of the canned fish industry also proceeded by leaps and bounds. For centuries, consumers inland had known nothing but the expensive freshwater fish, which was enjoyed only by the small minority who could afford it, as well as marinated or smoked "stock fish." But after 1880, the newly built

31. Grüttner, *Fleischversorgung*, p. 237.

railroads and the new techniques of refrigeration brought fresh ocean fish deep into the inland regions. The existing literature does not show exactly what the origins of the German fish canning industry were. It does seem certain, however, that the first attempts were made before the turn of the century. The first canned fish products were similar in taste to the traditional marinated and smoked products. It is said that in 1909 there were already four hundred fish canneries producing the cheap salt herring for the broad masses.[32] Canned fish was also imported. In 1913, the imports, consisting almost exclusively of sardines in oil, amounted to 3,500 tons. This was not very much because the domestic fisheries were protected from inexpensive foreign canned fish by high protective tariffs. When these tariffs were finally abolished after World War I, the imports rose sharply. In Germany, the large-scale production of canned fish products began about 1928–29, when herring and sprats in oil and tomato sauce, first developed in Norway, found a market. The traditional smoked fish industry declined correspondingly. While the per capita fish consumption in Germany has remained relatively constant (12 kg. in 1938, 11 kg. in 1965) the fish-processing industry has been able to increase its share of that market considerably since 1930.[33] The production of fancy foods—namely, the industrial canning of crabs, lobsters, sauces, mayonnaise, meat salads, condiments, and so on—also became part of this industrial branch. The world's first crab cannery was established in 1908 in the Gaimka Bay near Vladivostok, and "floating fish canneries" have existed since the 1920s.

The transition from artisanal to industrial mass production was made possible by close cooperation between science and technology. Various techniques of preservation had been tried out in the past, but it was not exactly known what happened during the process of preservation. The decisive understanding

---

32 Carl Winter, *Die deutsche Fischkonservenindustrie* (Jena, 1903); Edgar Lange, *Die Versorgung der grossstädtischen Bevölkerung mit frischen Nahrungsmitteln* (Leipzig, 1911).
33. Göben, *Fischwirtschaft*, p. 47.

of bacteria and their sterilization became available only through the research of Liebig, Pettenkofer, and Pasteur. These insights were the prerequisite for the full development of a modern food industry. Equally as important was the invention of the first autoclaves in Braunschweig (1873) and of the grooved lid in 1889. Soon thereafter the soldering machine was invented, so that laborious hand soldering was eliminated. All this coincided with the establishment of large-scale drying plants and with the development of refrigeration technology, so that the period between 1870 and 1914 marks the birth of the German canning industry. Between 1900 and 1914 the number of plants in the German Empire rose from 172 to 322. In the 1890s, the yearly production had not yet reached 1 million cans; in 1907, it reached about 35 million; and in 1913, 100 million kilo-size cans.[34] What had started as a stopgap for sailors and a luxury item for the rich had become an increasingly popular article of mass consumption.

However, the impact of canned foods on the standard of nutrition should not be exaggerated for the period before 1900. Traditional dietary habits were profoundly affected by them only at the very end of the century. Clearly, the central position was initially occupied by canned vegetables, which, as we pointed out, were the first items involved in this development. The greatest concentration of vegetable canning plants continued to be located in the Braunschweig–Hanover area, as well as in the adjoining regions of Saxony and Prussia. The *Altmark* (Lübeck and Hamburg) and Frankfurt-am-Main played a comparatively minor role. Only the mass production of sauerkraut, for which concrete silos, instead of the traditional smaller wooden barrels, were used as early as 1900 in Neuss on the Rhine, took place elsewhere. The Lower Rhine and Holstein became the centers of this new sauerkraut industry. Pickled cucumbers were industrially produced in the Neckar valley. The production of canned fruit, on the other hand, was long scat-

34. Herrmann, *Obst- und Gemüsekonservenindustrie*, p. 258.

tered among a number of smaller enterprises in southern Germany, since canned fruit was still considered a luxury item and therefore of less importance. After the turn of the century, this branch of the industry also settled in the Braunschweig area, which can thus be considered the cradle of the German canning industry. The industrial exploitation of mushrooms and wild berries remained the domain of the Bavarian forest. The growth in the capacity of the canning industry was considerable between 1900 and 1914. Before the war, the German Empire counted thirty-two canning factories, which produced an average of 1 million cans per year.[35] Obviously, their impact on the standard of nutrition must have been considerable. Their importance became even greater during the war, when canned vegetables were substituted for meat and fat. High demand brought about a deterioration of quality, which the government tried to check by law (May 26, 1916). Ever since then, all producers of canned foods must place their trademark on the can and adhere to minimum avoirdupois and minimum quality standards that are inspected by the health authorities.

Aside from the more conspicuous development of the canning industry, there were a number of lesser, but rather important, inventions to round out the picture of the nineteenth-century food industry. The Swiss mill owner Julius Maggi (1846–1912), native of the Kemp Valley, developed a ready-to-use "soup meal" made from vegetables, kitchen herbs, and other ingredients. He conceived his ideas as he watched the women and girls of his native region leaving the domestic hearth in order to work in factories. He realized that if women must work such long hours, they cannot spend much time on cooking. Since in the late nineteenth century it still took a whole morning to prepare a good soup, the Maggi cube was a welcome relief. Later he developed the Maggi condiments and founded a number of factories and companies in Singen-Hohentwiel, Bregenz, Vienna, Milan, and Paris. Karl-Heinrich Knorr, a native of the Braunschweig area who was originally in the legume busi-

35. Winkler, *Obst- und Gemüseverwertungsindustrie*, p. 257.

ness in Heilbronn, also realized that these products could be prepared industrially. In the 1870s, he and his two sons began to produce a variety of products from tapioca to green spelt and from pea meal to soup flour. He also seems to have introduced oatmeal flakes to the German market. The "dumpling king" Eckard, for his part, dedicated his life to the potato. In his search for a new technique of preservation, he produced potato flakes for the army during World War I. After the war, these were further developed into a product for making potato pancakes. The Eckard firm producing the ingredients for potato pancakes and dumplings took its name, "Pfanni," from the pan for frying potato pancakes and from a pert publicity girl named Fanni. In this manner, the potato dumpling was introduced into regions that had not known it traditionally. Finally, we must mention the industrial production of new substitutes for butter and coffee, namely, oleomargarine and Kathreiner's malt coffee (since 1892) and Franck's chicory coffee (since 1913), as well as the development of well-keeping lager beer.[36] All of these inventions are important aspects of industrialization and all of them have changed the standard of nutrition.

36. By comparison with other food items, the history of oleomargarine in the nineteenth century is remarkably well known, which is why it is not treated here in any great detail. Cf., however, the following works: Adolf Mayer, *Die Kunstbutter, ihre Fabrikation, ihr Gebrauchswerth, nebst Mitteln, ihren Vertrieb in seine Grenzen zurückzuweisen* (Heidelberg, 1884); C. Petersen, *Die Margarinefrage: Referat erstattet auf der Generalversammlung des Deutschen Milchwirtschaftlichen Vereins am 18. 2. 1895 zu Berlin* (Bremen, 1895); Louis Andes, *Kokosbutter und andere Kunstspeisefette* (Vienna and Leipzig, 1907); Heinrich Fränkel, *Der Kampf gegen die Margarine* (Weimar, 1894); C. Girard and J. Brevans, *La margarine et le beurre artificiel* (Paris, 1889); G. Hefter, *Technologie der Fette und Öle* (Berlin, 1910); Victor Lang, *Die Fabrikation von Kunstbutter, Sparbutter und Butterine* (Vienna, Budapest, and Leipzig, 1885); Ernst Feld, *Die deutsche Margarine-Industrie* (Hamburg, 1922); Gerhard Hülsbeck, "Die holländische Margarine-Industrie" (Ph.D. diss., Cologne, 1931); H. Limburg, *25 Jahre Vereinigung deutscher Margarinefabrikanten GmbH* (Cologne, 1921); H. van Voornfeld, *Die Margarine, ihre Herstellung, Vertrieb und volkswirtschaftliche Bedeutung mit Würdigung der rechtlichen Gesichtspunkte* (Trier, 1913); Franz W. Schlet, *Über Margarine, Bericht an das Central-Comité des Landwirtschaftlichen Vereins in Bayern* (Munich, 1895); Charles Wilson, *The History of Unilever* (London, 1954); Werner Schüttauf, *Die Margarine in Deutschland und in der Welt*, 4th ed. (Hamburg, 1962).

Changes in the Cost of Food as a Proportion of the Total Cost of Living

Changes in the cost of food to the working classes of the eighteenth and nineteenth centuries are difficult to gauge, not only because the sources are scanty and uneven and basic research inadequate, but also because incomes were not really comparable, prices fluctuated widely, and there were varying patterns of consumption. The results of the comparison between a very limited number of food budgets, such as was recently made by Lothar Schneider, can be cautiously formulated as follows:[37]

It is fairly certain that the cost of food in the investigated households of industrial and cottage workers between 1840 and 1880 took a much greater proportion of the total cost of living than is the case today, so that not much was left for superfluities (*freie Konsumspitze*) once the necessary outlays for food, rent, heating, and lighting were made. It appears that expenditures for food representing a large proportion of the cost of living are characteristic of industrially underdeveloped societies, especially in the lower social strata, a fact that can still be observed in present-day developing countries. According to the theory of marginal utility and to Engels' law, the proportion tends to decrease with more advanced industrialization and rising real wages. A very detailed analysis of cottage workers' household budgets between 1848 and 1878 shows that proportional outlays for food varied between 50 and 80 percent, depending on income, size of family, and aspirations. It should be added that a relatively high proportion of the food needs was still covered by domestic production. Perhaps too starkly, it could even be said that until the time of Bismarck's empire the food of the increasingly urbanized German factory worker still resembled the food of the rural cottage worker and the urban artisan to an astonishing degree. This conclusion, in any case, is suggested again and again by the household budgets that have come down to us.

On the other hand, this conclusion is not too surprising if we recall that at the beginning of any industrialization commuting

---

37. Schneider, *Arbeiterhaushalt*, pp. 51, 122 ff.

workers from the countryside play an important role in urban factories. In order to avoid the expensive eating places of the city, workers frequently ate only cold food they brought with them, or else their wives took a hot meal directly from the rural home to the factory. Furthermore, many "factory establishments," especially at the beginning, were located directly in the countryside because of the plentiful supply of cheap labor. In these cases, secularized monasteries and castles were particularly sought after, since they provided ample working space. As the cities expanded and distances between home and work became increasingly greater, factory workers liked to settle in rural communities and suburbs close to their factory. But even here it was still possible to engage in a kind of "mini-agriculture" for self-supply and supplementary income. With few exceptions, the cities of the nineteenth century were not yet the asphalt jungles, completely removed from the country, they were to become a few generations later. "Workers' colonies" near industrial centers always featured vegetable patches and fruit trees. Pigs, goats, doves, but especially rabbits and chickens, occasionally even beehives, were a common sight in the German workers' settlements well into the twentieth century. The famous "miner's cow" in the Ruhr district was an aspect of this supplementary agricultural activity that was carried on with the same intensity in Upper Silesia, Berlin, Saxony-Thüringia, and in the industrial areas of southern Germany. In this connection, the extensive garden colonies *(Schrebergärten)* at the outskirts of Berlin are particularly important. It is thus not surprising to see that for a long time the food of the urban wage earner remained in touch with the elements of his traditional agrarian existence. There was one group, however, that did not enjoy the support of this tradition. These were the "lodging boys" and "lodging girls," young people who could not afford their own room in the city and slept on a couch in a room heavy with the smells of cooking and laundry, in some cubby hole, or even in their landlord's bed. For the rest of their needs, they had to make do with what was available in cheap pubs or in workers' kitchens. From a nutritional point of view, this group was the first to be truly victimized by industrialization. The physical and moral misery of these "lodgers" was critically described and lamented again and again by contemporary social reformers, from clergymen and women's rights advocates to factory inspectors.

While it is true that factory workers had less and less opportunities for domestic production as time went on, increasingly placing them at the mercy of fluctuations in food prices, it must be kept in mind that, on the other hand, rising real wages improved the quality of their food.

According to Schneider's analysis, the average Prussian working-class family in the mid nineteenth century had to spend 58 percent of its income on the most important food staples, a figure that was reduced to 33 percent by 1913. Altogether, it can be estimated that before 1914 a factory worker had to spend between 50 and 70 percent of his total income on food, depending on the size of his family, his income, and his aspirations.[38] It appears that with the rise of real wages of the working classes the outlays for food increased in absolute terms because of the sharply rising food prices and the qualitative improvement in daily food, but that as a *proportion* of total expenditures, outlays for food decreased in favor of other purchases. Today, the average family in the Federal Republic of Germany spends only 35 percent of its income on food.[39] Only a detailed analysis of all existing household budgets of low-income families before World War I will be able to shed more

38. Cf. the very interesting graph "Cost of Living for a Mason's Family of Five in Berlin, ca. 1900," in Abel, *Agrarkrisen*, p. 230. The graph shows that this family spent 72.7 percent of its total income on food. The expenditures for food were distributed as follows: bread, 44.2 percent; animal products, 14.9 percent; other vegetable products, 11.5 percent; beverages, 2.1 percent. The expenditure for rent was 14.4 percent, for lighting and heating, 6.8 percent. Thus only 6.1 percent of the total income was available for clothing and other needs. The most exact data on the relationship between income and standard of living from the late Middle Ages to the present are still found in Abel, which is why it is necessary to cite them here once again. The whole complex of standard of living and income, particularly the relationship between income and diet, has been somewhat neglected in the present study in order to concentrate on the history of nutrition itself.

39. W. Wirths, W. Keller, and H. Kraut, "Work and Food," *Nutritio et Dieta* 8, no. 3–4 (1966).

light on this rather obscure chapter in the history of nutrition in Germany.

One thing, however, can already be considered certain: the outlays for food were essentially a function of the size of the family. The more numerous the family, the greater the part of the total income that was spent for food, and the greater also the proportion of the relatively cheaper vegetable foods. In the forty-four working-class households in Nürnberg analyzed by the union organizer Adolf Braun, the percentage of income spent for food was lowest in 2-person households; in 6–8 person households, it amounted to 50 percent; and in 7–10 person households, about 66 percent of the total income was spent for food.[40] The higher the total income of the family, the more would be spent for the highly nutritious animal proteins. The differences were considerable: within the sample of workers interviewed, the highest income group spent almost twice as much on animal foods as the lowest income group. The largest part of the caloric intake was always provided by bread (including flour) and potatoes; together with butter, these probably furnished 90 percent of the energy. It seems certain that the consumption of potatoes was highest in the lowest income groups. While the quantifiable relationships are still in great need of further study, these few examples already reveal that expenditures for food were a function of income and family size.

The Role of Food within the General Theory of Consumer Demand in Historical Perspective

Finally, we should try to draw even more abstract conclusions from the above findings. To this end, a number of economic and sociological theories must be critically examined.

As we pointed out earlier, today food no longer occupies first place in the normal household budget, since it requires only

---

40. Adolf Braun, *Haushaltsrechnungen Nürnberger Arbeiter* (Nuremberg, 1901), pp. 33, 63.

about one-third of the average income. In advanced industrial countries, we have almost forgotten that only at the beginning of this century, that is, two or three generations ago, the lower classes of the population had to spend as much as 40 to 70 percent of their income on food and drink, a figure that was probably even higher in earlier times. Outlays for clothes, housing, lighting, hygiene, not to mention cultural pursuits, played a very modest role indeed by present-day standards. Because of the great importance of food in the general circulation of goods and in the distribution of income, political economists have long been interested in this particular topic.

In 1853, Herman Heinrich Gossens formulated his theory of marginal utility for the consumption side of the economy in his book *Gesetze des menschlichen Verkehrs*. Like the Englishman William Stanley Jevons and the Austrian theoreticians of value who elaborated his theories, Gossens frequently used examples taken from the area of food consumption to demonstrate his general theory of demand when he examined the intensity of desire for specific kinds of goods in relation to their availability. Thus it was shown that the desire for wheat will be very strong when only limited stocks are available, but that desire will decrease as soon as there is enough wheat, not only for ample human consumption, but for the fattening of fowl, the making of spirits, and even the feeding of parrots. No doubt the thesis that the so-called marginal utility conditions the intensity of demand for a given product at a given time is correct in the main and explains minor differences in demand as well as certain fluctuations in the value of the product. If we apply the theory of marginal utility to the total change in nutritional standards in Germany over the nineteenth century, however, even a preliminary investigation makes it clear that changes in the underlying structures of demand—the more subtle gradations in the various kinds of needs, changes and differentiations in the value attributed to foodstuffs according to time and place or to social class—cannot really be explained by it. The change in the standard of nutrition in Germany has very little or nothing to do with individual feelings of pleasure or displeasure, but rather with changes in supply, cost of production, distribution, techniques of production and preservation, and finally, with factors related to social milieu.

Like all other attempts to base the interpretation of total demand on a theory of consumption, the theory of marginal utility had its usefulness for explaining the circulation of goods and the distribution of income, but it is also an almost classic illustration of the fact that fundamental changes in human food consumption can never be fully explained by a single-cause theory. Like many others, this theory is an important tool for attacking a mass of raw data, but by itself it cannot hope to establish historical truths. Gossens's laws are a means for taking a fresh look at the course of history. But it turns out that this will not provide historical orders of magnitude. It does not even indicate the approximate direction taken by the changes in food consumption. Individual feelings of pleasure or displeasure with their food and drink have not been a decisive factor for most consumers of the nineteenth centuy. Level of income, habit, the symbolic connotations of certain foods and beverages, and so on, have no doubt been much more influential in shaping the pattern of consumption. The theory of marginal utility does not explain to the social and economic historian why certain nutritional needs have remained relatively stable throughout the ages while others have changed. By taking a fresh look at the traditional categories, Lujo Brentano's brilliant theory of needs has provided many psychologically, sociologically, and even historically valuable insights and in the process refuted a great deal of nonsense in the older literature of classical political economy. But he too was unable to establish a general law of food consumption.

The fact that general theories of consumer demand are more or less useless to historians of nutrition is certainly related to their particular way of looking at things. They are not interested in the fluctuating demands of an imagined stable market, but on the contrary, in change and causes of change and in the great turning points of economic and social processes. They must study the actual course of history, even if its individual steps are revealed only piecemeal.

Nonetheless, the historian of nutrition owes another, and vastly more important, insight to theoretical political economy. For that science teaches us that food is always a twofold historical quantity. It appears (1) as the sum total of a desired and consumed product, and (2) as the quantity present in the market at any given time. The quantity of food present in the market will be proportionally smaller as domestic production is more extensive, so that many foods do not even appear in the market. As we pointed out, there are no statistics about domestic production, but individual examples suggest that it must have been considerable. The fact that in 1860 two-thirds of all bread was still baked at home in North Germany (in France the figure is one-half as late as 1900) is one such indication. Since only the surpluses of the agricultural producers were in the market, we must conclude that not all real consumers appeared as buyers in the food sector. Fluctuations in the price of foodstuffs therefore affected a relatively smaller group than they do today. Because of the high incidence of domestic production, the price fluctuations so painstakingly traced by Wilhelm Abel and other agrarian historians provide only an incomplete picture of the actual food situation. Price statisitics do give important indications about incomes, but they do not say enough about the development of the standard of living in general. Until the late nineteenth century, domestic production of foodstuffs was extensive in most parts of Germany, even in urban areas. It was only later that food prices assumed the importance for an analysis of the nutritional situation that they have today. Even so, we must not overlook the fact that, given a fairly well developed system of money and credit, the domestic production was, in a certain sense, a value within the market, since the foods produced and consumed, but not sold, constituted a kind of market reserve that can be expressed in terms of money. Historians must constantly keep in mind that their analysis of these phenomena is largely based on various kinds of estimates and that they can not rely solely on the demand registered in the market, but must also take into account the totality of real demand.

The general theory of consumer demand yields a further interesting insight: in the food sector, as in others, only part of the market was arranged in such a way that the producer, on the one hand, and the consuming household, on the other—that is, two entirely different functions—were directly confronting each other in the economic process. As in all sectors of economic demand, some of the consumers were in reality producers (and/or middlemen) as well. The food industry, for example, acted as a consumer when dealing with the farmer but as producer when dealing with wholesale or retail merchants. Especially in the history of nutrition, producer and consumer are not always clearly distinguishable, since they frequently assumed each other's role. This fact complicates the whole problem of food prices even further.

While in the last analysis producer and consumer remain the decisive factors in the working of the market, it must be kept in mind that the interchange of these functions was particularly prevalent and confusing in the food sector. Until late in the nineteenth century, most households in Germany were always potential sellers of foodstuffs because of the already mentioned high incidence of domestic production. As we pointed out above, such direct fulfillment of food needs had become less and less prevalent over the centuries. With the development of the monetary economy and the division of labor, increasing numbers of entrepreneurs and middlemen inserted themselves into the process of food production and distribution. On the whole, of course, this development must be considered progress, for specialists in a particular area are in a much better position to judge demand for food and drink than the individual consumer. The food trade owed its very existence to the fact that it could deal with all markets at any given time better than individual producers and consumers. Thus the situation in the nineteenth century was fundamentally different from earlier times, for the butcher or baker in the medieval guild system made his living primarily because he owned a privilege, not because he knew how to take advantage of a free market. The industrial production of food and its distribution by means of numerous middlemen led to abuses, to monopolies, and to the exploitation of the unprotected consumer. For the food-producing entrepreneur and the distributing middleman were not primarily interested in providing optimal supply to the entire population, but rather in their own profit, which was always influenced by competing supplies and by general demand. Momentary disposition of producer and middleman, conditions of credit, discounts, price-fixing, and similar factors later also began to play a role. As far as can be ascertained, the effect of these factors on the changing nutritional habits of the nineteenth century has been studied only partially and in insufficient depth.

Steps in the Development of the Standard of Nutrition and Sociological Types of Nutrition

A general survey of the history of human nutrition as far as it is known to us makes it abundantly clear that over the centuries it has become increasingly easy to satisfy the need for food. The diet of primitive man must have been extremely imperfect, if only because he did not cultivate grain or keep domestic animals. He neither knew bread nor butter, neither salt, sugar, beer, or milk.

Only slowly did he learn to amass provisions, to keep them, and to use them efficiently. Fishing, the culture of grain and tuberous plants, the domestication of wild animals, the use of milk and the making of butter, as well as the salting, smoking, and drying of meat, mark the second great step in the history of human nutrition. No doubt the most difficult problem was solved at this point. More abundant supplies enabled man to evolve a completely new economic, social, and political life, created the conditions to sustain a marked increase in population, and paved the way for higher forms of civilization and technology. It is true, of course, that difficulties in food supply were never completely solved, especially since it initially proved impossible to produce grain and meat on large tracts and/or in mass quantities. Such production required the development of entirely new techniques. The problem of mass production of foods and their shipping over long distances was solved only by the industrialization of the nineteenth century, marking a third step in the development of the standard of nutrition.

Hunger and thirst, taste and aesthetic sensibility, as well as ethical and religious norms, have determined the demand for food over thousands of years. Ignorance of the composition of individual foodstuffs and the organic processes by which the human body makes use of food also has frequently misdirected consumption habits. As far as can be ascertained, entire tribes, nations, and social classes have long existed on faulty diets, misunderstood the nutritional value of certain foods, and misinterpreted the effects of certain luxuries and stimulants. Many of these errors were recognized only by the new nutritional sciences of the nineteenth century. This knowledge, however, did not immediately reach the broad masses.

Economic necessities certainly did shape nutritional behavior in Germany in the direction of greater rationality, but irrational motives continued to play a part. As the workers' household budgets have shown, expenditures for food were, in many cases, uneconomical and conditioned by emotion. As we have pointed out, the idea of "good food" was often mistakenly equated with that of "abundant food." The important thing was to give the stomach as much as it could hold. In particular, not enough milk, fruit, vegetables, and fish were consumed. This was the beginning of the age of the calorie, but not of vitamins. The failure to adapt the traditional agrarian food habits to the changed industrial environment was certainly an obstacle to proper nutrition. The worker's wife who came to the Ruhr area from East Prussia about 1880 must have found it difficult to adapt the cooking skills she had learned from her mother or grandmother in a rural household to the exigencies of an urban household in an industrial environment. The robust country-style food designed to be eaten by men who did heavy work in the fields proved to be physiologically "system-incongruent," as it were, in an industrial situation. It has rightly been pointed out that a comparison of the cooking skills in the various social strata shows that such skills seem to be directly related to definite social structures. The fact that workers' daughters were absent from the home all day long did not develop any particular skills in food preparation, and therefore were unable to manage a household in the traditional fashion was an incentive to the food industry to fill this new need by producing canned goods. It thus becomes apparent that industrialization influenced nutritional behavior, but that the latter, in turn, also stimulated the development of industry. In this manner, seemingly minor differences in food habits assume great sociological and historical significance.

The history of nutrition shows that there were many mistakes and false starts, but also great progress. Improvements in gardening and farming, the development of the food industry, refinement in the art of preserving and cooking, more and more different kinds of food in the market, on the whole, made for a better, more varied, and even more aesthetically pleasing diet. Specialized diets for the various professions and activities were developed quite early. Even in the nineteenth century, the lower social classes participated, at least to some extent, in the progress of nutrition, even though many of their desires for a sufficient and appropriate diet remained unfulfilled. Various consumption statistics and household budgets suggest that the following types of diet existed in the nineteenth century:

1. The freely chosen diet of the upper classes
2. The diet of the urban artisan, the lower-level employee and civil servant, and the highly skilled worker
3. The diet of the independent farmer, fisherman, day laborer, and farmhand
4. The diet of the rural cottage worker and artisan who engage in domestic food production
5. The diet of the unskilled urban wage laborer who is solely dependent on money

In this scheme, type 3 must be considered the oldest type of diet from which all others have developed. This sociological classification of diets seems to have been established originally by a German follower of Le Play, Gottlieb Schnapper-Arndt, who based them on his analysis of household budgets.[41] With the modifications added in the present study, these sociological types still seem to be useful as a structuring device. Subsequent research could, of course, subdivide them further. Alfred Grotjahn, who postulated similar types of diets in his work, felt that the nineteenth century was characterized by the disintegration of older, usually local types of diet. Type 3 ate a much more monotonous and less palatable diet than type 5, though the latter still had many shortcomings. According to his research as a physician practicing around 1900, the traditional rural type of diet, especially that of the rural workers, had deteriorated because people now had to market everything that could be sold from their domestic production, so that they consumed less eggs, milk, chicken, pork, and fats than before. Thus their predominantly starchy diet of flour and potatoes became more insufficient and inappropriate than ever. By contrast, Grotjahn claimed that the better-paid skilled workers were coming closer to the freely chosen diet of the upper classes, as indicated by their increased consumption of meat, eggs, and milk. But the masses of ordinary, unskilled industrial workers were caught in the transition from the traditional rough, monotonous, and simple peasant diet to the more refined and varied diet of the well-to-do. In this manner, the lower classes were taken out of the age-old agricultural economy and the social order implied in such a system. Yet, by the end of the nineteenth century, the new way of life based on a money economy was not yet satisfactorily established either. Only today, two generations later, can we see that this transition is nearing its completion. The oldest rural type of diet seems to be well-nigh extinct, since the food industry is now offering its products in the most remote village. The average worker's diet is so close to the freely chosen, varied diet of the upper classes that day-to-day food consumption can hardly be considered a social indicator any longer. By and large, the transition to an industrialized type of diet is complete. While there are still certain regional variations, significant social differences in diet no longer exist.

41. Gottlieb Schnapper-Arndt, *Sozialstatistik* (Leipzig, 1912), p. 406.

Selected Bibliography

Introductions to "Food in History"

Braudel, Fernand. *Capitalism and Material Life, 1400–1800.* New York: Harper & Row, 1973.

Furnas, C. C., and Furnas, C. M. *Man, Bread and Destiny.* New York: Reynal & Hitchcock, 1937.

English Food Habits

Barker, T. C.; McKenzie, J. C.; and Yudkin, J. *Our Changing Fare: Two Hundred Years of British Food Habits.* London: MacGibbon & Kee, 1966.

Drummond, J. C., and Wilbraham, A. *The Englishman's Food: Five Centuries of English Diet.* London: Jonathan Cape, 1939, 1958.

The Irish Famine

Connell, K. H. "The Potato in Ireland." *Past and Present,* no. 23 (1962), pp. 57–70.

Woodham-Smith, Cecil. *The Great Hunger: Ireland, 1845–1849.* London: Hamish Hamilton, Ltd., 1962.

French, German, and Other European Food Habits

Hémardinquer, J.-J. *Pour une histoire de l'alimentation.* Cahiers des Annales no. 28. Paris: Colin, 1970. This volume contains thirty-one articles on dietary history from the sixteenth to the nineteenth century and includes such varied areas as Venice, Geneva, Valladolid, Tuscany, Poland, Russia, the Balkans, Scandinavia, England, the Maghreb, Canada, and numerous regions of France. The bibliography also cites sixteen more articles published by the *Annales:E.S.C.* since 1961, including F. Braudel's "Bulletin No. 1," launching the "attack" on *l'histoire alimentaire.*

Aron, J.-P. *Essai sur la sensibilité alimentaire à Paris au 19ᵉ siècle.* Cahiers des Annales no. 25. Paris: Colin, 1967.

LeRoy Ladurie, E. *Times of Feast, Times of Famine: A History of Climate since the Year 1000.* Garden City, N.Y.: Doubleday, 1971.

Stouff, L. *Ravitaillement et alimentation en Provence aux XIVᵉ et XVᵉ siècles.* Paris: Mouton, 1970.

Teuteberg, H. J., and Wiegelmann, G. *Der Wandel der Nahrungsgewohnheiten unter dem Einfluss der Industrialisierung.* Göttingen: Vandenhoek & Ruprecht, 1972. This is a pioneer work in German social and economic history and one of the first to deal comprehensively with working-class diet. It ranks with Hémardinquer and Drummond-Wilbraham as a basic work in the field.

Popular Works Useful to the History of Dietary Habits

Ellwanger, G. H. *Pleasures of the Table: An Account of Gastronomy from Ancient Days to Present Times.* New York: Singing Tree Press, 1902. Reprint, Detroit, 1969.

Pullar, P. *Consuming Passions: Being an Historic Inquiry into Certain English Appetites.* Boston and Toronto: Little, Brown, 1971.

Tannahill, Ray. *Food in History.* New York: Stein & Day, 1923.